CARDIOLOGY RESEARCH AND CLINICAL DEVELOPMENTS

CONGENITAL HEART DISEASE

FROM DIAGNOSIS TO TREATMENT

CARDIOLOGY RESEARCH AND CLINICAL DEVELOPMENTS

Additional books and e-books in this series can be found on Nova's website under the Series tab.

CARDIOLOGY RESEARCH AND CLINICAL DEVELOPMENTS

CONGENITAL HEART DISEASE

FROM DIAGNOSIS TO TREATMENT

CURTIS GIGUÈRE
EDITOR

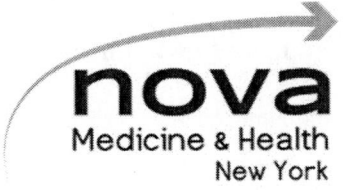

Copyright © 2020 by Nova Science Publishers, Inc.

All rights reserved. No part of this book may be reproduced, stored in a retrieval system or transmitted in any form or by any means: electronic, electrostatic, magnetic, tape, mechanical photocopying, recording or otherwise without the written permission of the Publisher.

We have partnered with Copyright Clearance Center to make it easy for you to obtain permissions to reuse content from this publication. Simply navigate to this publication's page on Nova's website and locate the "Get Permission" button below the title description. This button is linked directly to the title's permission page on copyright.com. Alternatively, you can visit copyright.com and search by title, ISBN, or ISSN.

For further questions about using the service on copyright.com, please contact:
Copyright Clearance Center
Phone: +1-(978) 750-8400   Fax: +1-(978) 750-4470   E-mail: info@copyright.com.

NOTICE TO THE READER

The Publisher has taken reasonable care in the preparation of this book, but makes no expressed or implied warranty of any kind and assumes no responsibility for any errors or omissions. No liability is assumed for incidental or consequential damages in connection with or arising out of information contained in this book. The Publisher shall not be liable for any special, consequential, or exemplary damages resulting, in whole or in part, from the readers' use of, or reliance upon, this material. Any parts of this book based on government reports are so indicated and copyright is claimed for those parts to the extent applicable to compilations of such works.

Independent verification should be sought for any data, advice or recommendations contained in this book. In addition, no responsibility is assumed by the Publisher for any injury and/or damage to persons or property arising from any methods, products, instructions, ideas or otherwise contained in this publication.

This publication is designed to provide accurate and authoritative information with regard to the subject matter covered herein. It is sold with the clear understanding that the Publisher is not engaged in rendering legal or any other professional services. If legal or any other expert assistance is required, the services of a competent person should be sought. FROM A DECLARATION OF PARTICIPANTS JOINTLY ADOPTED BY A COMMITTEE OF THE AMERICAN BAR ASSOCIATION AND A COMMITTEE OF PUBLISHERS.

Additional color graphics may be available in the e-book version of this book.

Library of Congress Cataloging-in-Publication Data

ISBN: 978-1-53616-674-3
Library of Congress Control Number:2019954055

Published by Nova Science Publishers, Inc. † New York

CONTENTS

Preface		vii
Chapter 1	Congenital Heart Disease and Pregnancy *Maeve K Hopkins and Jeffrey A. Kuller*	1
Chapter 2	Pregnancy Considerations in Women with Congenital Heart Disease *Brian Z. Druyan and Martina L. Badell*	23
Chapter 3	Cardiac Resynchronization Therapy in Adults with Congenital Heart Disease: Current State and Future Perspectives *Rohit K. Kharbanda, Ad J. J. C. Bogers and Natasja M. S. de Groot*	53
Chapter 4	Types, Presentation, and Management of Atrial Septal Defects in Adults *Samantha Whitwell, Frank Han, Michael McMullan and William Campbell*	75
Chapter 5	State of the Liver in Children with Congenital Heart Disease *M. P. Lymarenko*	91

Chapter 6	High Altitude and Congenital Heart Disease in Andean Highlands Populations: The Case of Ecuador *Fabricio González-Andrade,* *Stephanie Michelena, Daniel Echeverría Espinosa* *and Gabriela Aguinaga Romero*	**107**
Index		**177**
Related Nova Publishers		**181**

PREFACE

Congenital Heart Disease: From Diagnosis to Treatment opens with a review of the most common forms of congenital heart disease in pregnancy, outlines preconception counseling, discusses the associated morbidity and mortality of each lesion, and reviews current recommendations for the management of congenital heart disease in pregnancy.

Women with congenital heart disease represent over 50% of patients with cardiac disease in pregnancy today. Formerly characterized by high rates of maternal morbidity and mortality, the authors explore how advancements in medical management and surgical intervention are responsible for increasing numbers of women with congenital heart defects experiencing safe and successful pregnancies.

Additionally, the authors discuss cardiac resynchronization therapy in adults with congenital heart disease. Treatment in the setting of heart failure is challenging due to heterogeneity of the underlying anatomy and physiology, surgical scars, residual shunts and valvular dysfunction. Since donor hearts are scarce, worldwide interest has increased for the application of cardiac resynchronization therapy in this relatively young population.

This compilation goes on to discuss the four different types of atrial septal defects, categorized based on location and embryological development. While bicuspid aortic valve is the most common congenital heart anomaly in adults, atrial septal defects are not far behind, accounting for 10-15% of congenital heart disease.

In the penultimate study, the authors focus on the state of the liver in children with congenital heart disease and chronic heart failure. Congenital heart disease represented: ventricular septal defect – in 26,7% of patients, secondary atrial septal defect – in 24,4% of children, a double discharge of the main vessels of the right ventricle – in 15,6% of patients, common atrioventricular canal – at 15,6% of children, tetralogy of Fallot – at 11,1% of patients, etc.

The concluding study reviews the effects of high altitude effects on congenital heart disease in the Andean region, and in Ecuador as a study case. High-altitude hypoxia presents numerous challenges to human health, survival, and reproduction because of decreased oxygen availability brought on by lowered barometric pressure at high elevations.

Chapter 1 - Congenital heart disease (CHD) refers to a "gross structural abnormality of the heart or intrathoracic great vessels that is actually or potentially of functional significance". Congenital heart disease is the most common congenital anomaly and makes up approximately one-third of congenital defects. Due to advanced surgical and medical therapy for CHD, more women with CHD are reaching childbearing age, representing a unique challenge to obstetric providers. With advances, women with CHD are more frequently reaching childbearing age and conceiving. Many women with CHD can have successful pregnancies, although there are a few conditions that represent significant maternal risk such that pregnancy is considered contraindicated. Appropriate obstetric care for women with CHD requires a knowledge of cardiac physiology in pregnancy, the anatomy of CHD and repaired CHD, and coordinated care from cardiology and maternal-fetal medicine specialists. This chapter reviews the most common forms of CHD in pregnancy, outlines preconception counseling, discusses the associated morbidity and mortality of each lesion, and reviews current recommendations for management of CHD in pregnancy.

Chapter 2 - Women with congenital heart disease represent over fifty-percent of patients with cardiac disease in pregnancy today. Formerly characterized byhigh rates of maternal morbidity and mortality, advancements in medical management and surgical intervention are responsible for increasing numbers of women with congenital heart defects experiencing safe and successful pregnancies. However women with congenital heart disease who become pregnant do remain at higher risk for adverse pregnancy outcomes and cardiac complications during pregnancy. Consequently, it is imperative that healthcare providers caring for these women and their babies are well informed about the best practices and guidelines to providing care. As more women with congenital heart disease pursue pregnancy, a collaborative multidisciplinary approach to the management of these patients and their pregnancies is critical to achieving optimal perinatal outcomes and minimizing morbidity.

Chapter 3 - Advances in therapy have resulted in an ever-increasing population of grown-ups with congenital heart disease (GUCH), also called adults with congenital heart disease (CHD), in whom sudden cardiac death and progressive heart failure are predominant causes of mortality. Treatment of adults with CHD in the setting of heart failure is challenging due to heterogeneity of the underlying anatomy and physiology, surgical scars, residual shunts and valvular dysfunction. Since donor hearts are scarce, worldwide interest has increased to apply cardiac resynchronization therapy (CRT) in this relatively young population. CRT is an established therapy for heart failure in patients with idiopathic or ischemic heart disease and electromechanical dyssynchronous ventricles. European and American guidelines provide specific indications for CRT in these patient groups, however these criteria are not directly applicable to patients with CHD. Since there are no randomized controlled trials in patients with CHD, the recommendations for CRT in this patient population is extrapolated from relatively small retrospective studies. Results from current retrospective studies are promising, however there are some major limitations. Relatively small number of patients in a heterogeneous group (including both pediatrics and adults) and a limited follow-up duration are important shortcomings of these studies, precluding long term outcomes. Moreover, patients with cardiomyopathies and congenital atrioventricular block are often included as patients with 'CHD' leading to results representing the outcome in a mixed population. The current GUCH guidelines do not provide indications for CRT as evidence supporting CRT has thus far been limited to case reports and retrospective studies in a heterogeneous patient population with different underlying cardiac defects. For the challenging systemic RV population, the guidelines state that CRT is still experimental. In these patients, the benefits of CRT are less clear. In the following chapter, current experience of CRT in adults with CHD is summarized and future perspectives are discussed.

Chapter 4 - There are four different types of atrial septal defects (ASDs) categorized based on location and embryological development. While the bicuspid aortic valve is the most common congenital heart anomaly in adults, ASDs are not far behind, accounting for 10-15% of congenital heart disease [5, 6]. They also account for approximately 100 of 100 000 live births in the current era of echocardiography. While some familial conditions, such as Holt-Oram syndrome are associated with ASDs, the inheritance pattern is mostly unknown. Other syndromes associated with atrial septal defects include Down Syndrome, Ellis van Creveld Syndrome, and Digeorge Syndrome. Within the spectrum of atrial septal defects, the secundum subtype is the most common (~75%), followed by the ostium primum, sinus venosus, and coronary sinus atrial septal defects.

Chapter 5 - Congenital heart disease (CHD) – one of the most common congenital anomalies in children (30% of all congenital malformations); in terms of frequency of occurrence, it ranks third after congenital pathology of the musculoskeletal system and central nervous system.

It should be noted that in diseases of the heart, including congenital heart disease, the liver is affected due to an acute or chronic increase in central venous pressure, as well as a decrease in cardiac output. The phenomena of stagnation, necrosis, fibrosis, less often cirrhosis, which may exist separately, but are often combined depending on the clinical situation, are usually observed. To refer to these disorders, a number of authors suggest the term «cardiogenic liver».

In the medical literature there are very few reports on the state of the liver, cholestatic disorders in children with congenital heart disease. Most publications concern Alagille syndrome.

The purpose of the authors' research was to study the state of the liver in children with congenital heart disease and chronic heart failure. The authors observed 45 children. Congenital heart disease represented: ventricular septal defect – in 26,7% of patients, secondary atrial septal defect – in 24,4% of children, a double discharge of the main vessels of the right ventricle – in 15,6% of patients, common atrioventricular canal – at 15,6% of children, tetralogy of Fallot – at 11,1% of patients, etc. Combined congenital heart disease were diagnosed in 17,8% of children. Hepatosplenomegaly without liver dysfunction was found in 75,6% of patients. In all cases, enlargement of the liver associated with hemodynamic compromise and venous stagnation of blood in it.

Chapter 6 - It is estimated that there are around 83 million people living at high altitudes; over 2500 meters above sea level (masl) worldwide. Andean (highlands), Tibetan, and Ethiopian populations have lived under chronic hypoxia conditions for thousands of years. From those, groups who have been residing there for over a millennium in three high-altitude zones of the globe are the Sherpa and Ayurveda (Qinghai-Tibetan Plateau), the Kichwa and Aymara highlanders (Andean Altiplano), and the Ethiopian Amhara and Oromo highlanders (the Semien Plateau in Ethiopia). For them, the adaptive and maladaptive changes have occurred at the genomic and physiological levels. In Ecuador, for example, most of the capital cities are located at altitudes above 2500 masl.

High-altitude hypoxia presents numerous challenges to human health, survival, and reproduction due to the decreased oxygen availability brought on by lowered barometric pressure at high elevations. Changes in pulmonary function, arterial oxygen saturation (SaO_2) hemoglobin concentration, and maternal physiology during pregnancy among others have permitted high-altitude natives to thrive in the harsh conditions. Most common adaptative changes involves ventilation rates, hypoxic ventilatory response, elevated arterial oxygen saturation, elevated hemoglobin concentration, and elevated birth weight.

Despite these adaptations, it seems that some diseases are more commonly observed within these populations. For instance, the prevalence of Congenital Heart Disease (CHD) in newborns at high altitude is about 20 times higher than at low altitude. High altitude is an environmental risk factor for CHD, especially patent ductus arteriosus (PDA). By 18 months of age, about 60% of left to right shunts remain unclosed. Atrial Septal Defect (ASD), Ventricular Septal Defect (VSD) and Left Ventricular Outflow tract obstruction LVOTO are show frequently at high altitude.

Researchers have tried to explain the role of high altitude on CHD for over 60 years, describing different mechanisms, including embryonic tissue hypoxia. The increase frequency of CHD at high altitudes clearly suggest a leading role for environmental mechanisms mediated by low atmospheric pressure and the persistence of pulmonary hypertension after birth. Screening newborn children for CHD) mostly focus on critical CHD using pulse oximetry.

This is a review of high altitude adaptation, and its effects on CHD focused in the Andean region, and in Ecuador as a study case.

In: Congenital Heart Disease
Editor: Curtis Giguère

ISBN: 978-1-53616-674-3
© 2020 Nova Science Publishers, Inc.

Chapter 1

CONGENITAL HEART DISEASE AND PREGNANCY

Maeve K Hopkins[1] and Jeffrey A. Kuller[2]
[1]Maternal Fetal Medicine, University of Pennsyvlania,
Philadelphia, PA, US
[2]Maternal Fetal Medicine, Duke University Hospital,
Durham, NC, US

ABSTRACT

Congenital heart disease (CHD) refers to a "gross structural abnormality of the heart or intrathoracic great vessels that is actually or potentially of functional significance" [1]. Congenital heart disease is the most common congenital anomaly and makes up approximately one-third of congenital defects [2]. Due to advanced surgical and medical therapy for CHD, more women with CHD are reaching childbearing age, representing a unique challenge to obstetric providers. With advances, women with CHD are more frequently reaching childbearing age and conceiving. Many women with CHD can have successful pregnancies, although there are a few conditions that represent significant maternal risk such that pregnancy is considered contraindicated. Appropriate obstetric care for women with CHD requires a knowledge of cardiac physiology in pregnancy, the anatomy of CHD and repaired CHD, and coordinated care from cardiology and maternal-fetal medicine specialists. This chapter reviews the most common forms of CHD in pregnancy, outlines preconception counseling, discusses the associated morbidity and mortality of each lesion, and reviews current recommendations for management of CHD in pregnancy.

Keywords: pregnancy, congenital heart disease, birth defects, high-risk pregnancy

INTRODUCTION

Leonardo da Vinci may have depicted the first image of a congenital heart defect. He drew a partial anomalous pulmonary venous connection of the right pulmonary veins to the right atrium. The first reported surgical management of CHD was ligation of a patent ductus arteriosus (PDA) by Gross and Hubbard [3] in 1939 at Boston Children's Hospital. This ushered in an era of pediatric cardiovascular surgery for CHD. In 1944, surgeons in Sweden successfully repaired an aortic coarctation (AoC) [4], and surgeons in the United States reported a procedure to anastomose the subclavian artery to the pulmonary artery to palliate cyanotic congenital heart defects called a Blalock-Taussig shunt [5]. Since the mid-20th century, advances in surgical and medical management of CHD have led to dramatic increases in survival and quality of life of patients with CHD. Due to advances, more women of child-bearing age are becoming pregnant with CHD.

In terms of prevalence, congenital heart disease is the most common major congenital anomaly. In one large review, the prevalence of CHD was estimated to be 9.1 per 1000 live births, which equates to 1.35 million newborns with CHD born worldwide every year. The prevalence varies by geographic region, with rates highest in Asia, followed by Europe and lowest in North America. The most common subtype is ventricular septal defect (VSD, 34%), followed by atrial septal defect (ASD, 13%) [6-7].

PHYSIOLOGY

Normal pregnancy involves extensive cardiovascular adaptation. In a normal pregnancy, cardiac output increases by 30% to 50%, primarily through decreased systemic vascular resistance and low-resistance placental blood flow. This results in reduced mean arterial pressure, which triggers an increase in plasma blood volume, heart rate, and stroke volume. Heart rate and cardiac output increase rapidly in the late first trimester and continue to increase until approximately 25 weeks of gestation, and plasma volume reaches its peak at 32 weeks of gestation. In the third trimester, stroke volume declines as pressure on the vena cava increases with uterine size [8-12].

During labor, uterine contraction pain leads to higher levels of circulating catecholamines, causing increased heart rate and cardiac contractility. Additionally, preload increases due uterine contractions, which results in an additional 300 to 500 mL of venous blood returning to the heart. The net effect is an approximately 30% increase in cardiac output during labor. In the second stage of labor, Valsalva maneuvers cause a decrease in venous return and can result in marked fluctuations in central venous pressure [13].

Immediately postpartum, the uterus involutes and caval compression is released, leading to autotransfusion of around 500 mL of uteroplacental blood back into the circulation. This increases venous return and increases preload. As a result, cardiac output increases by approximately 60% to 80% immediately after delivery, thus offsetting the effects of bleeding. Beginning at 48 hours after delivery, diuresis and natriuresis occur, and blood pressure and blood volume return to prepregnancy levels by around 10 days postpartum. Heart rate remains elevated for 24 hours after delivery and then declines to prepregnancy ranges within 10 days. Notably, the extravascular fluid mobilization that occurs between 2 and 4 days postpartum increases the risk of pulmonary edema [14].

Congenital Heart Lesions in Pregnancy

Ventricular Septal Defect (VSD)

VSDs are the most common congenital heart defects in childhood and make up approximately 25% of cases of CHD. The prevalence of VSDs in the adult population is lower, as there is a high rate of spontaneous closure of small defects during childhood. Ventricular septal defects result from a delay in closure of the interventricular septum beyond the first 7 weeks of gestation. Ventricular septal defects are classified based on the location of the defect within the ventricular septum as perimembranous, supracristal (infundibular), muscular, and inlet. The most common type is the perimembranous VSD (approximately 80%).

The natural history and clinical course of patients with a VSD depend on the size of the defect and the pulmonary vascular resistance. Typically, asymptomatic adult patients with repaired or isolated, small (<25% of the aortic annulus diameter) VSDs do not require surgical closure and are expected to have normal long-term outcome. In contrast, adults with large (>75% aortic annulus) unrepaired VSDs usually develop left ventricular failure and pulmonary hypertension, progressing to Eisenmenger syndrome [14].

The diagnosis of VSD often occurs in childhood after detection of a systolic heart murmur, typically located at the left lower sternal border. Smaller defects have louder associated murmurs and may be accompanied by a palpable thrill. If significant volume overload is present, the precordial impulse may be displaced laterally, and a diastolic flow murmur across the mitral valve may be appreciated. Patients with Eisenmenger syndrome may be noted to have cyanosis, clubbing, and a right ventricular (RV) heave.

In addition to the physical examination, evaluation may include electrocardiogram, which is typically normal in patients with a small, restrictive VSD. If a significant shunt is present, there may be evidence of atrial enlargement (broad, notched P wave) and left ventricular dilation (deep Q waves and tall R wave in the left precordial leads) on ECG. Chest x-ray may show enlarged pulmonary arteries or increased pulmonary vascularity, as well as an enlarged cardiac border. Echocardiogram is the diagnostic test of choice to delineate the size, location, and functional effect of the lesion. In cases of large VSD or in cases of concern for hemodynamic compromise, the work up may include cardiac catheterization.

Many VSDs undergo spontaneous regression in size or even closure during early childhood and do not require intervention. In addition, small VSDs with minimal shunting do not require closure. Large VSDs often lead to significant left to-right shunting and LV volume overload, resulting in symptoms and requiring medical therapy and/or repair early in life. Transcatheter closure of VSDs was introduced in 1987 by Lock and colleagues [15] and provides an alternative to surgery.

Because large VSDs are often detected and repaired early in life, most unrepaired VSDs seen in pregnant women are small. Women with small or moderately sized restrictive VSDs, without pulmonary hypertension, and with normal left ventricular function do not have an increased risk of complications related to pregnancy. Women with large VSDs associated with significant shunting are at increased risk of left ventricular dysfunction, heart failure, and arrhythmias during pregnancy. Patients with significant pulmonary hypertension are at risk of complications regardless of whether the VSD has been repaired. In women with isolated VSDs that have been successfully repaired, pregnancy is generally well tolerated. However, combined atrioventricular septal defects (AVSDs) lead to more pregnancy complications.

Atrial Septal Defects (ASDs)

ASD is a common congenital heart defect and accounts for 7% of CHD. There are 5 types of ASDs: primum, secondum, coronary sinus, superior sinus venosus, and inferior sinus venosus. The ostium primum defects occur when there is a deficiency of endocardial cushion tissue and result in a defect in the inferior atrial septum just superior to the inflow portion of the atrioventricular (AV) valves. Primum defects are often associated with AV valve abnormalities. Secundum ASDs result from tissue defects within the oval fossa. Sinus venosus defects result from deficiency of in-folding of the atrial wall adjacent to the vena cava. Superior sinus venosus defects are often associated with anomalous pulmonary venous connections. Coronary sinus defects develop when there is a deficiency of the wall between the coronary sinus and the left atrium. This defect can be associated with a persistent left-sided superior vena cava.

Most children and even young adults with ASDs are asymptomatic. Left-toright shunting can increase over time, however, and can ultimately lead to progressive RV volume overload, RV hypertrophy, and, rarely, pulmonary hypertension. Patients with a primum ASD and associated AV valvular defects may be symptomatic earlier than individuals with an uncomplicated secundum ASD. Patients with secundum ASDs may develop shortness of breath or palpitations as the right ventricle begins to dilate or decline in function.

Possible physical examination findings in patients with unrepaired ASD include a wide and fixed splitting of the second heart sound, a systolic pulmonary flow murmur, and a mid-diastolic flow murmur across the tricuspid valve. Cyanosis is rare but may be present in patients with a very large defect or in the presence of other associated congenital lesions.

In addition to physical examination, the evaluation may include ECG, which may show right-axis deviation, incomplete right bundle-branch block, and evidence of RV hypertrophy, first-degree AV block, and left superior axis in primum defects. Chest x-ray may show enlargement of the right ventricle and pulmonary artery dilation; however, a normal chest radiograph does not rule out ASD. Echocardiogram is again the diagnostic study of choice and can show the size of the defect and estimate the amount of shunting, as well as assess for anomalous pulmonary venous return. If visualization is inadequate, transesophogeal echocardiogram, magnetic resonance imaging, or even cardiac catheterization may be indicated.

Atrial septal defects that result in symptoms, significant left-to-right shunting, or changes in RV size or function should be repaired. Defects can be closed surgically with a pericardial patch or percutaneously in selected patients. Patients with pulmonary hypertension have a poorer prognosis and may not benefit from surgical correction, as closure of the ASD could exacerbate symptoms.

Pregnancy is hemodynamically well tolerated in most patients with uncomplicated ASDs. In women with ASDs complicated by significant pulmonary hypertension, pregnancy is contraindicated. In a retrospective review, 4.3% of pregnant women with ASDs experienced significant arrhythmias, and 3% experienced a decrease in New York Heart Association (NYHA) functional status during pregnancy. Patients with unrepaired ASDs had a higher risk of preeclampsia (odds ratio, 3.54; 95% confidence interval, 1.26–9.98) and having fetuses who were small for gestational age [16]. In patients with combined AVSD, as can be seen in association with septum primum defects, cardiac complications occurred in 40% of pregnancies in a large retrospective review. Patients with CHD are often assessed based on their NYHA functional classification, which is a I–IV scale based on cardiac symptoms and functional status. In this study, 23% of patients experienced postpartum persistence of NYHA class deterioration, and 19% experienced arrhythmias during pregnancy. Although studies are limited, this study indicates that in women with AVSD pregnancy may not be well tolerated, and there is a risk for worsening cardiac status after delivery [17].

Left Ventricular Outflw Obstruction: Aortic Stenosis and Aortic Coarctation

Aortic Stenosis

Aortic stenosis (AS) is the most common valvular heart disease seen in the developed world and accounts for 3% to 6% of cases of CHD. Stenosis results from a fusion of the valve commissures, which results in rigidity of the valve leaflets and resulting obstruction. This stenosis can occur in both bicuspid and tricuspid aortic valves. Obstruction can worsen over time, particularly with calcification of the valve. Progressive left ventricular outflow obstruction leads to left ventricular strain and hypertrophy and can ultimately lead to left ventricular dysfunction.

On physical examination, a systolic ejection murmur with carotid radiation can be audible. A single or paradoxically split-second heart sound and delayed carotid upstroke are consistent with severe AS.

In addition to physical examination, evaluation may include ECG findings related to left ventricular hypertrophy such as increased voltage of the QRS complex. Chest x-ray shows typically normal size, but dilation of the ascending aorta may be present, particularly in patients with bicuspid aortic valve. Echocardiogram provides information on the severity of stenosis, as well as ventricular size and function. Cardiac catheterization may be used to assess the severity of stenosis when noninvasive testing is inconclusive.

Management outside of pregnancy depends on the severity of symptoms, as well as the degree of valve obstruction. The aortic valve gradient, or pressure across the aortic valve, can be calculated by echocardiogram using Bernoulli equation. The severity of AS is characterized based on velocity of blood flow and pressure gradient across the valve, as well as aortic valve area. Once symptoms develop, surgical or transcatheter intervention should be considered. In selected young patients with congenital bicuspid aortic valve, balloon aortic valvuloplasty can be considered.

Procedural intervention for asymptomatic AS is not routinely recommended. Surgical options for treatment include valve replacement with mechanical or biologic valves, or the Ross procedure in children and younger patients. The Ross procedure involves removing the pulmonary valve and proximal pulmonary artery and replacing this at the aortic root.

Complications in pregnancy increase with severity of AS. Severe AS in pregnancy is associated with increased rates of hospitalization, congestive heart failure (CHF), and supraventricular tachycardia. Neonatal risks include small for gestational age and prematurity [18]. Asymptomatic women with mild to moderate AS are more likely to tolerate pregnancy well if left ventricular function and exercise capacity are normal. Women with symptomatic or severe AS often tolerate pregnancy poorly. Patients who are symptomatic or who have severe AS prior to pregnancy are advised to delay conception until after surgical correction. If the patient is symptomatic before the end of the first trimester, pregnancy termination or repair should be considered. Aortic valve replacement and palliative aortic balloon valvuloplasty have been successfully performed during pregnancy, although there are associated maternal and fetal risks [19]. Women with bicuspid aortic valves and associated dilatation of the ascending aorta should be monitored carefully for increases in aortic size by echocardiogram.

Aortic Coarctation

Aortic coarctation (AoC) is a discrete narrowing of the proximal thoracic aorta and occurs in 6% to 8% cases of CHD. The true etiology of AoC is unknown, and theories include postnatal constriction of aberrant ductal tissue and intrauterine alterations of blood flow through the aortic arch. Aortic coarctation is classified as preductal or postductal and occurs in 1 per 12,000 live births. Aortic coarctation is often associated with other CHDs, such as bicuspid aortic valve, PDA, VSD, or mitral valve abnormalities. A peak pressure gradient of 20 mm Hg or greater across the coarctation is clinically significant.

Severe AoC can be associated with VSD and/or bicuspid aortic valve and often presents in infancy with symptoms of CHF. In adults, AoC is associated with upper body hypertension. Physical exam may show a blood pressure decrease between upper and lower extremities, weak and delayed lower-extremity pulses, and a systolic murmur at the left sternal border.

The workup of AoC varies greatly based on the severity of the coarctation and includes the electrocardiogram, which may show LVH. Chest radiograph may show dilated aorta, inferior rib notching, or distortion of the appearance of the ribs due to enlarged collateral blood vessels. Noninvasive testing includes echocardiogram or magnetic resonance imaging (MRI)/computed tomography angiogram. MRI is the preferred imaging study. Echocardiogram requires suprasternal views to identify the site of narrowing, and Doppler evaluation of the descending aorta can reveal an abnormal flow pattern. Invasive testing with cardiac catheterization or angiography may be required in patients with complex coarctation or associated valvular lesions.

Aortic coarctation associated with obstructive left ventricular lesions often carry a poor prognosis and require surgical intervention in infancy. However, mild, isolated coarctation can go unrecognized into adulthood and can be associated with increased risk of ischemic heart disease and cerebral vascular accidents.

Outside of pregnancy, aortic coarctation can be treated with placement of a pericardial patch, surgical repair, balloon angioplasty, or stenting. The incidence of recoarctation after surgical repair ranges from 8% to 44%, and patients may require recurrent treatment. Patients with upper-extremity/lower-extremity pressure gradients of less than 20 to 30 mm Hg should be followed up to assess increasing pressure gradient, aneurysm formation, or development of collateral blood flow [12].

In terms of pregnancy, one retrospective review of pregnant women with AoC (both repaired and unrepaired), demonstrated that major cardiovascular complications in pregnancy were rare, although coarctation was associated with an increased rate of pregnancy-associated hypertension [20]. In patients with unrepaired AoC and enlargement of the proximal aorta, the diagnosis of aortic dissection should be considered; this diagnosis may necessitate urgent attention and cesarean delivery [21].

In a large study of 118 pregnancies in patients affected by AoC, 9% miscarried, 3% delivered preterm, 30% developed hypertension during pregnancy, and 73% of these women had hemodynamically significant coarctation during that time [20]. Women with coarctation and Turner syndrome are considered at higher risk for hypertensive and cardiovascular complications during pregnancy.

Right Ventricular Outflow Obstruction

Pulmonic Stenosis

Pulmonic stenosis leads to anatomic obstruction of flow from the right ventricle to the pulmonary arterial vasculature and most often occurs in the setting of Tetraology of Fallot (TOF). Isolated pulmonic valvular stenosis (90%) typically results from fusion of the valve commissures, dysplastic valves (such as a small valve annulus in Noonan syndrome), or a bicuspid valve.

Physical examination may reveal a crescendo-decrescendo systolic murmur at the left upper sternal border, which would be more audible in pregnancy due to higher volume/flow. A pulmonary ejection click that decreases during inspiration may be heard.

In addition to a physical examination, evaluation includes ECG, which may show right-axis deviation or RV strain in severe obstruction, but most often is normal. Chest x-ray may show dilatation of the left and main pulmonary arteries. Echocardiogram can show valve morphology, in addition to predicted pressure gradient across the RV outflow tract, as well as the presence and degree of RV hypertrophy or tricuspid regurgitation.

In a large retrospective review of 81 completed pregnancies in women affected by pulmonic stenosis, there were a relatively high number of hypertension-related disorders (15%, including 5% with preeclampsia). In this study, the premature delivery rate was 17%, and 3.7% of women experienced thromboembolic events [22]. In general, although RV outflow obstruction can lead to RV hypertrophy and may increase the risk of volume overload during pregnancy, most reports indicate that patients with isolated PS generally tolerate pregnancy well, particularly in the absence of hypertensive disorders.

In the presence of normal cardiac output, the RV-PA pressure gradient determines management of isolated PS. Most patients with an RV systolic pressure or pulmonary valve gradient between 50 and 79 mm Hg require intervention. Balloon valvuloplasty and surgical valvotomy can relieve the obstruction. Patients with a gradient less than 50 mm who are asymptomatic can generally be monitored for symptoms without intervention during pregnancy.

Tetralogy of Fallot

Tetralogy of Fallot is the most common cyanotic CHD. During embryologic development, anterior/superior infundibular septal displacement leads to the tetrad of VSD, overriding aorta, RV hypertrophy, and pulmonic outflow obstruction (PS). This leads to decreased pulmonary blood flow from the right ventricle and increased right-to-left shunting across the VSD. In the setting of associated severe PS, the right-to-left shunting across the VSD can result in significant cyanosis.

Tetralogy of Fallot is most often diagnosed in infancy and physical exam is associated with a prominent systolic murmur, cyanosis and possibly cyanotic spells. The vast majority of patients undergo repair during childhood in order to patch the VSD and relieve the obstruction of the RV outflow tract. Pulmonary valve insufficiency may subsequently develop.

Physical exam in the adult patient with corrected Tetralogy of Fallot can vary but may include prior sternotomy site, and findings consistent with residual pulmonic stenosis or VSD. Evaluation of the adult patient with history of TOF repair may include ECG, which likely shows right-axis deviation and RV hypertrophy. On chest radiograph, classically the heart is of normal size, but may have the shape of a boot due to RV hypertrophy and diminished pulmonary artery shadow. Echocardiogram can provide information regarding degree of RV outlet obstruction and valvular function. Cardiac catheterization may be necessary to assess pulmonary arteries prior to surgical repair, and if persistent RV outflow obstruction is noted after surgical correction, catheterization can determine the site of obstruction. Treatment of TOF is surgical, consisting of VSD closure and relief of RV outflow obstruction. Total correction is often performed in the first year of life if the pulmonary arteries are of adequate size.

Most studies report generally favorable pregnancy outcomes in women with repaired TOF and hemodynamic stability entering pregnancy. Some risks during pregnancy include fetal growth restriction or low birth weight and premature delivery [23–25]. In the event of pulmonic valve insufficiency, the volume load of pregnancy can result in RV overload, enlargement, and right-sided heart failure. Studies suggest that patients with significant pulmonic regurgitation and RV dysfunction have the highest risk of pregnancy complications, and these patients should be counseled appropriately prior to becoming pregnant [23].

In a large study of 112 pregnancies in women with TOF, 27% of pregnancies resulted in miscarriage. Unrepaired TOF ($P = 0.05$) and morphologic pulmonary artery abnormality ($P = 0.03$) were independently predictive of lower infant birth weight. Six patients had cardiovascular complications during pregnancy: supraventricular tachycardia in 2 patients, heart failure in 2 patients, pulmonary embolism in a patient with pulmonary hypertension, and progressive RV dilation in a patient with severe pulmonic regurgitation. Five infants (6%) had congenital anomalies.

Management in pregnancy depends on the severity of pulmonic regurgitation and RV function. Khairy et al. [23] found that the presence of severe PI was an independent predictor of primary cardiac events during pregnancy, with an odds ratio of 4.6. The most common cardiac event in this study was heart failure that responded to medical therapy without need for further intervention. There were no maternal deaths. Therefore, in summary, the data suggest that although women with TOF and severe pulmonary regurgitation are at risk of right-sided heart failure and arrhythmia, they respond well to medical therapy, with no other likely adverse outcomes [23].

Transposition of the Great Vessels

In patients with dextro-TGA, there is ventriculoarterial discordance: systemic venous return enters the right atrium and right ventricle and exits the aorta, whereas pulmonary venous return flows from the pulmonary veins to the left atrium, left ventricle, and pulmonary artery. This results in severe cyanosis typically manifesting in the first 1-2 days of life, because there is inadequate mixing of the 2 circulations to allow adequate oxygenation. Adult patients will have had surgical correction either by the arterial switch procedure, which establishes the normal relationship between the ventricles and the great arteries (common after 1991), or by an atrial switch procedure, which maintains the morphologic right ventricle as the systemic ventricle. Prior to the atrial switch repair, many patients were treated surgically with a Mustard-Senning procedure. This procedure creates a baffle, or conduit, between the 2 atria to allow for oxygenation of blood.

In the neonatal period, physical exam shows evere cyanosis, although infants with TGA and a VSD may present later in childhood as the VSD allows mixing of blood and increased oxygenation. In addition to physical examination, evaluation includes ECG, which may reveal RV hypertrophy, right-axis deviation, and possible sinus bradycardia or sick sinus syndrome (rhythm disturbances indicating dysfunction of the sinoatrial node). Chest radiograph may reveal RV cardiac silhouette and slight increase in cardiothoracic ratio. Echocardiogram will have characteristic appearance after atrial switch correction and can be used to monitor pulmonary and systemic pathways.

Studies have shown varying rates of both maternal and obstetric complications. Patients who have undergone the atrial switch procedure are at risk of systolic dysfunction and inadequate contractility in response to the physiologic changes in pregnancy. Prior surgical correction may also predispose to arrhythmias.

A large study of a national registry examined outcomes of 49 completed pregnancies with repaired transposition. The most common cardiovascular complication was arrhythmia (22%). Heart failure occurred in 2 pregnancies, and worsening of NYHA class occurred in 17 pregnancies. The decline in NYHA class persisted for 1 year after pregnancy in 8% of patients. There were no maternal deaths. Pregnancy complications included preeclampsia (10.2%) and pregnancy induced hypertension (8.2%), premature rupture of membranes (14.3%), preterm labor (24.4%), premature delivery (31.4%), small for gestational age (21.6%), and thromboembolic complications (4.1%) [26].

One study compared women with TGA atrial switch repair in childhood and examined cardiac outcomes in those who became pregnant versus nonpregnant control subjects. No deaths occurred; however, events such as arrhythmias, thromboembolic events, and baffle issues were common in both groups: 62% in pregnant patients and 53% in nonpregnant control subjects, P = 0.736. Worsening of ventricular function was also similar in both groups: 29% of pregnant patients and 27% of control subjects (P = 0.899). Worsening tricuspid regurgitation was more common among pregnant patients (52%) than control subjects (0), P < 0.001. In terms of pregnancy outcomes in this study, 32% of patients were delivered because of cardiac deterioration, and 38% of infants were preterm, and 38% were small for gestational age [27]. Another study followed 24 pregnancies in 15 women with previous Mustard-Senning operation to correct TGA. Two pregnancies ended in first-trimester miscarriage. Although 5 pregnancies had obstetric complications (1 patient with gestation diabetes, 1 patient with hypertension, 1 patient with placenta increta, and 2 patients with preterm labor), there were no severe cardiac complications in pregnancy or in the postpartum period [28].

Management of women with TGA during pregnancy depends on the original repair. For pregnant women who have undergone an atrial switch procedure and therefore have a systemic right ventricle, close observation for signs of heart failure or volume overload is recommended.

Preconception Counseling

Preconception counseling is essential in women with a history of CHD. Appropriate counseling should include comprehensive medical and surgical history, physical examination, 12-lead electrocardiogram, and echocardiogram, including Doppler studies. In patients with history of impaired or questionable functional capacity, an exercise test, preferably with measurement of oxygen consumption, is useful for an objective assessment of functional classification. The anticipated risk of pregnancy based on the evaluation should be discussed with the patient and her family by both the cardiologist and the obstetrician in conjunction with consultation from a maternal-fetal medicine specialist. In patients with severe disease, relative or absolute contraindications to pregnancy, or NYHA class III or IV, the risk of severe maternal morbidity or even mortality should be discussed.

In anticipation of pregnancy, medications with potential harm to the fetus such as ACE inhibitors should generally be discontinued and replaced with safer options [29]. The risk of pregnancy can be discussed and generally predicted based on the NYHA functional class, which is highly predictive of maternal and fetal outcome [30]. In addition, the patient with CHD should be counseled that their offspring carries an increased risk of CHD, ranging from 3% to 5% [31].

Bacterial Endocarditis Prophylaxis

Prophylaxis for bacterial endocarditis is recommended in women at highest risk of endocarditis when undergoing dental procedures involving gingival manipulation or perforation of oral mucosa. Eligible patients include those with prosthetic cardiac valves; a prior personal history of infective endocarditis; unrepaired cyanotic CHD, including palliative shunts and conduits; repair of CHD with prosthetic material in the past 6 months; and history of repaired CHD with residual defects adjacent to a prosthesis. Prophylaxis is also recommended in women with a history of a heart transplant with existing valvular dysfunction.

Although no formal recommendation exists, the American College of Obstetricians and Gynecologists recommends consideration of prophylactic antibiotics for vaginal delivery in patients with cyanotic cardiac disease, prosthetic valves, or both. In patients with the aforementioned high-risk conditions who have an established infection such as chorioamnionitis, treatment of the active infection is prioritized, whereas additional prophylactic treatment for endocarditis is not recommended [32].

Anticoagulation

Certain cardiac conditions may confer increased risk of thrombus formation. Since pregnancy is a thrombogenic state, anticoagulation may be considered or indicated in women with CHD and pregnancy. Particularly women with arrhythmias such as atrial fibrillation may require anticoagulation. In women with arrhythmias such as atrial fibrillation at risk of stroke, weight-based low molecular weight heparin (Lovenox) can be used for anticoagulation [35]. Given the potential teratogenic effect of warfarin and limited information on other oral anticoagulants such as Xa inhibitors, lovenox is generally the preferred anticoagulant during pregnancy.

In addition to arrhythmias, anticoagulation (either prophylactic or therapeutic), may be considered in cases of reduced ejection fraction, complicated repairs such as Fontan circulation, or other complex CHD. The discussion of indication for and type of anticoagulation should be interdisciplinary and involve a specialized cardiologist, maternal-fetal medicine specialist, and discussion with the patient regarding risks and benefits during pregnancy.

Contraindications to Pregnancy

Few absolute contraindications to pregnancy exist, but include the following:

- Severe pulmonary hypertension, defined as PApressure equal to or greater than 75%systemic pressure
- Severe obstructive lesion (aortic/mitral stenosis, HOCM, coarctation)
- Systemic ventricular systolic dysfunction, defined as class III or IV CHF
- Marfan aortopathy with dilated aortic root equal to or greater than 40 mm.

In addition to Marfan aortopathy, women with monosomy X (Turner Syndrome), although often subfertile or infertile, can conceive, particularly in the era of assisted reproductive technology. Women with monosomy X have approximately a 2% maternal death rate, a 1% to 2% risk of aortic dissection, and a 1% risk of worsening CHD [34]. In women Turner Syndrome with a significant cardiac defect or an enlarged aortic size index, pregnancy is contraindicated due to a higher rate of aortic dissection in pregnancy [36].

Other risk factors for adverse cardiac events during pregnancy (defined as maternal heart failure, arrhythmia, stroke, or maternal death) that are not absolute contraindications include maternal cyanosis, LV systolic dysfunction (defined as LVejection fraction ≤40%), left-sided heart obstruction (peak gradient ≥40 mm Hg), and history of prior severe arrhythmias or cardiac events (e.g., arrhythmia, stroke, pulmonary edema). If a woman presents in pregnancy with absolute contraindications, termination should be discussed, and in some situations, surgical correction of cardiac lesion during pregnancy could be considered.

REFERENCES

[1] Mitchell SC, Korones SB, Berendes HW. Congenital heart disease in 56,109 births incidence and natural history. *Circulation*. 1971;43:323–332.

[2] Dolk H, Loane M, Garne E, et al. Congenital heart defects in Europe: prevalenc and perinatal mortality, 2000 to 2005. *Circulation*. 2011;123:841–849.

[3] Gross RE, Hubbard JP. Surgical ligation of a patent ductus arteriosus. Report of first successful case. By Robert E. Gross and John P. Hubbard. *JAMA*. 1939;112:729–731.

[4] Crafoord C, Nylin G. Congenital coarctation of the aorta and its surgical treatment. *J Thorac Surg*. 1945;14:347–361.

[5] Blalock A, Taussig HB. The surgical treatment of malformations of the heart: in which there is pulmonary stenosis or pulmonary atresia. *JAMA*. 1945;128:189–202.

[6] Van der Linde D, Konings EE, SlagerMA, et al. Birth prevalence of congenital heart disease worldwide: a systematic review and meta-analysis. *J Am Coll Cardiol*. 2011;58:2241–2247.

[7] Hoffman JI, Kaplan S. The incidence of congenital heart disease. *J AmColl Cardiol*. 2002;39:1890–1900.

[8] Meah VL, Cockcroft JR, Backx K, et al. Cardiac output and related haemodynamics during pregnancy: a series of metaanalyses. *Heart*. 2016;102:518–526.

[9] Sanghavi M, Rutherford JD. Cardiovascular physiology of pregnancy. *Circulation*. 2014;130:1003–1008.

[10] Carbillon L, Uzan M, Uzan S. Pregnancy, vascular tone and maternal hemodynamics: a crucial adaptation. *Obstet Gynecol Surv*. 2000;55:574–581.

[11] Van Oppen AC, van der Tweel I, Alsbach GP, et al. A longitudinal study of maternal hemodynamics during normal pregnancy. *Obstet Gynecol*. 1996;88:40–46.

[12] Gersony WM, Rosenbaum MS. Congenital Heart Disease in Adults. New York: McGraw-Hill; 2002.

[13] Ouzounian JG, Elkayam U. Physiologic changes during normal pregnancy and delivery. *Cardiol Clin.* 2012;30:317–329.
[14] Gatzoulis, et al. Diagnosis and Management of Adult Congenital Heart Disease. Philadelphia, PA: Saunders; 2011.
[15] Lock JE, Block PC, McKay RG, et al. Transcatheter closure of ventricular septal defects. *Circulation.* 1988;78:361–368.
[16] Yap SC, Drenthen W, Meijboom FJ, et al. Comparison of pregnancy outcome in women with repaired versus unrepaired atrial septal defect. *BJOG.* 2009;116:1593–1601.
[17] Drenthen W, Pieper PG, van der Tuuk K, et al. Cardiac complications relating to pregnancy and recurrence of disease in the offspring of women with atrioventricular septal defects. *Eur Heart J.* 2005;26:2581–2587.
[18] Orwat S, Diller GP, vanHagen IM, et al. Risk of pregnancy inmoderate and severe aortic stenosis: from the Multinational ROPAC Registry. *J AmColl Cardiol.* 2016;68:1727–1737.
[19] Bernal JM, Miralles PJ. Cardiac surgerywith cardiopulmonary bypass during pregnancy. *Obstet Gynecol Surv.* 1986;41:1–6.
[20] Beauchesne LM, Connolly HM, Ammash NM, et al. Coarctation of the aorta: outcome of pregnancy. *J Am Coll Cardiol.* 2001;38:1728–1733.
[21] Task Force on cardiovascular disease during pregnancy of the European Society of Cardiology. *Eur Heart J.* 2003;24:761–781.
[22] Drenthen W, Pieper PG, Roos-Hesselink JW, et al. Non-cardiac complications during pregnancy in women with isolated congenital pulmonary valvar stenosis. *Heart.* 2006;92:1838–1843.
[23] Khairy P, Ouyang DW, Fernandes SM, et al. Pregnancy outcomes in women with congenital heart disease. *Circulation.* 2006;113:517–524.
[24] Veldtman GR, Connolly HM, Grogan M, et al. Outcomes of pregnancy in women with tetralogy of Fallot. *J Am Coll Cardiol.*2004;44:174–180.
[25] Presbitero P, Somerville J, Stone S, et al. Pregnancy in cyanotic congenital heart disease. Outcome of mother and fetus. *Circulation.*1994;89:2673–2676.

[26] Drenthen W, Pieper PG, Ploeg M, et al. Risk of complications during pregnancy after Senning or Mustard (atrial) repair of complete transposition of the great arteries. *Eur Heart J.* 2005;26:2588–2595.

[27] Cataldo S, DoohanM, Rice K, et al. Pregnancy following Mustard or Senning correction of transposition of the great arteries: a retrospective study. *BJOG.* 2016;123:807–812.

[28] Lipczyńska M, Szymański P, Trojnarska O, et al. Pregnancy in women with complete transposition of the great arteries following the atrial switch procedure. A study from three of the largest adult congenital heart disease centers in Poland. *J Matern Fetal Neonatal Med.* 2017;30:563–567.

[29] Elkayam U, Bitar F. Valvular heart disease and pregnancy part I: native valves. *J Am Coll Cardiol.* 2005;46:223–230.

[30] Siu SC, Sermer M, Colman JM, et al. Prospective multicenter study of pregnancy outcomes in women with heart disease. *Circulation.* 2001;104:515–521.

[31] Nora JJ, Nora AH. Recurrence risks in children having one parent with a congenital heart disease. *Circulation.* 1976;53:701–702.

[32] American College of Obstetricians and Gynecologists. ACOG Practice Bulletin No. 120: use of prophylactic antibiotics in labor and delivery. *Obstet Gynecol.* 2011;117:1472–1483.

[33] Earing MG, Webb GD. Congenital heart disease and pregnancy: maternal and fetal risks. *Clin Perinatol.* 2005;32: 913–919.

[34] Chevalier N, Letur H, Lelannou D, et al. Materno-fetal cardiovascular complications in Turner syndrome after oocyte donation: insufficient prepregnancy screening and pregnancy follow-up are associated with poor outcome. *J Clin Endocrinol Metab.* 2011 Feb;96(2):E260-7.

[35] American College of Cardiology, Recommended Doses of Anticoagulant/Antithrombotic Therapies for Patients with Atrial Fibrillation. https://www.acc.org/tools-and-practice-support/clinical-toolkits/atrial-fibrillation-afib/anticoagulant-dosing-table. Accessed 8/27/19.

[36] Practice Committee of the American Society for Reproductive Medicine 2012. Increased maternal cardiovascular mortality associated with pregnancy in women with Turner syndrome. *Fertil Steril.*97:282-284.

In: Congenital Heart Disease
Editor: Curtis Giguère

ISBN: 978-1-53616-674-3
© 2020 Nova Science Publishers, Inc.

Chapter 2

PREGNANCY CONSIDERATIONS IN WOMEN WITH CONGENITAL HEART DISEASE

Brian Z. Druyan, MD and Martina L. Badell*, MD
Emory University School of Medicine, Department of Gynecology and Obstetrics, Division of Maternal Fetal Medicine, Atlanta, Georgia, US

ABSTRACT

Women with congenital heart disease represent over fifty-percent of patients with cardiac disease in pregnancy today. Formerly characterized by high rates of maternal morbidity and mortality, advancements in medical management and surgical intervention are responsible for increasing numbers of women with congenital heart defects experiencing safe and successful pregnancies. However women with congenital heart disease who become pregnant do remain at higher risk for adverse pregnancy outcomes and cardiac complications during pregnancy. Consequently, it is imperative that healthcare providers caring for these women and their babies are well informed about the best practices and guidelines to providing care. As more women with congenital heart disease pursue pregnancy, a collaborative multidisciplinary approach to the management

---

* Corresponding Author's Email: mbadell@emory.edu.

of these patients and their pregnancies is critical to achieving optimal perinatal outcomes and minimizing morbidity.

INTRODUCTION

Congenital heart disease [CHD] represents the most common congenital anomaly. Innovative medical, surgical, and diagnostic techniques continue to decrease the mortality and morbidity associated with congenital heart disease [3, 14, 10]. Today, women born with CHDcan expect to live fuller lives and usually reach reproductive age [3, 8]. Consequently, there is now a growing demographic of women bearing children with managed congenital heart defects [3, 14, 10]. Thus, composing a comprehensive set of guidelines and information to promote optimal outcomes and safety for this unique population of women is imperative. This chapter seeks to define this population and outline the most contemporary recommendations for the care and management of these women as they pursue childbirth.

BACKGROUND

Approximately 1-4% of live-births in the Unites States today are complicated by cardiovascular disease [17, 6]. At the same time, 20% of non-obstetric deaths in pregnancy are consequences of cardiac events [13]. As rates of diabetes, hypertension, obesity, and the average age of childbearing increase, the rates of cardiac disease and cardiac related complications are also expected to rise [8, 17]. Of the utmost concern are the unique challenges posed by the rapidly growing cohort of pregnant women with congenital heart disease.

There are currently an estimated 1.4 million adults living with CHD in the United States and nearly half of those individuals are women above the age of 18 [8, 17]. Estimates project continued growth of this population at a rate of 5% annually [17]. Not only is the number of women born with CHD reaching reproductive age rising, but the number of deliveries among this cohort is likewise increasing. In less than one decade, from 1998 to 2007, the number of deliveries among patients with CHD increased by more than 30% [17].

Although many of these women may tolerate pregnancy well, research suggests that this growing demographic experiences substantially higher rates of maternal and fetal morbidity, cardiovascular complications, and comorbid conditions relative to the general population [17]. Data suggests that upwards of 12% of women with CHD can anticipate a cardiac complication at some point during their pregnancy. Generally, the risks are directly proportional to the severity of their underlying disease [17]. Consequently, the more intricate and complex care required by these patients accounts for longer hospitalizations and increased costs that place an additional burden on the healthcare system.

In the coming years, as more women with CHD become mothers, clinicians and health systems alike must generate guidelines and protocols aimed at providing these patients with the specialized care and treatments they need to optimize their outcomes.

PHYSIOLOGIC CHANGES OF PREGNANCY

Pregnancy is characterized by the marked adaptation of the maternal body to both support and sustain the development and growth of the fetus as well prepare the mother to withstand the physical demands of labor and delivery (Table 1).

The cardiovascular system, in particular, undergoes a series of profound alterations with important consequences for cardiac health- especially in regards to patients with pre-existing cardiac disease and CHD. Starting shortly after conception, maternal blood volume begins to expand and ushers in the characteristic hypervolemic state of pregnancy. Increases in both plasma volume and red blood cell mass combine to expand blood volume by approximately 40-45% in the gravid woman [3, 16]. Owing to the comparatively larger rise in plasma volume relative to red blood cell mass, maternal blood experiences a physiologic hemodilution [16]. This disproportionate expansion results in the physiologic anemia of pregnancy seen in the second and third trimesters [3, 16].

As plasma volume and red blood cell mass expand early in pregnancy, so, too, does cardiac output. Soon after conception, cardiac output begins to increase steadily through 24 weeks of gestation. Maternal cardiac output surges to 30-50% above pre-pregnancy levels as a function of increasing heart rate and stroke volume [3, 16]. Additionally, cardiac output becomes significantly more sensitive to positional changes from 20 weeks gestation onward as a result of the mass effect of the gravid uterus on the inferior vena cava and pelvic veins [3, 16]. Supine and lithotomy positions can contribute to precipitous declines in cardiac output by upwards of 25-30% at term [3].

Similarly, underlying an increase in cardiac output, heart-rate also experiences a gradual rise throughout pregnancy. By the third trimester, maternal heart-rate is typically 10-20 bpm above pre-pregnancy levels and is the predominant force driving the overall increase in maternal cardiac output later in pregnancy [3, 16]. In conjunction with increases in cardiac rhythm, pregnancy contributes to a decreased threshold for arrhythmias including premature atrial and ventricular beats as well as reentrant supraventricular tachycardias [3]. This is particularly pertinent given the proclivity of many women with CHD to develop arrhythmias arising from their respective lesions.

To contend with the volume expansion in pregnancy, the systemic vascular resistance and pulmonary vascular resistance both experience a decline. Systemic vasodilation, resulting from progestogenic effects, leads to as much as a 30% decline in systemic vascular resistance as early as 5 weeks into pregnancy [3, 16]. The decrease in SVR correspondingly decreases both preload and afterload contributing to significant alterations in the hemodynamic state of the gravid woman [3, 17]. Similarly, the pulmonary vascular resistance drops by nearly a quarter compared to pregestational values by the 8th week of gestation in order to adapt to the nearly 50% increase in pulmonary circulation [16].

The alterations in the cardiovascular system during pregnancy are numerous. All of these changes can precipitate significant adverse outcomes and predispose vulnerable patients, like those with CHD, to a maternal and or fetal complications as they progress through pregnancy.

Table 1. Physiologic changes in pregnancy

Physiologic Component	Degree of Change in Pregnancy
Cardiac Output	40-50% increase
Stroke Volume	30% increase
Heart Rate	20-25% increase
Intravascular Volume	40-45% increase
Systemic Vascular Resistance	20% decrease
Blood Pressure	Decreases in first and second trimesters Return to baseline in third trimester
Oxygen Consumption	30 - 40% increase
Left ventricular wall mass	Increases
Chamber sizes of the heart	Increase in size of all 4 chambers

"Cardiovascular Physiology of Pregnancy." Circulation. https://www.ahajournals.org/doi/full/10.1161/circulationaha.114.009029.

PRECONCEPTION COUNSELING

Integral to optimizing the safety and wellbeing of women with CHD who desire to become pregnant is preconception counseling. Undergoing a comprehensive clinical evaluation by a multidisciplinary team of providers is important to determine any anticipated complications and possible threats to the mother and developing fetus [3, 15]. Additionally, the implicit risks to the developing fetus, including the risk of inheriting a cardiac anomaly, warrants discussion before pursuing pregnancy. The Modified World Health Organization Pregnancy Risk Classification for Women with Congenital Heart Disease is one of the classification systems that can be used both prior to and during pregnancy to help determine the risk of adverse cardiac events during pregnancy.

Maternal Assessment

The foundation of individualized risk stratification for women with CHD involves a detailed cardiovascular exam and a global inventory of the patient's medical history [9]. Determining the specific type of cardiac defect, the history of surgical repairs, extent of residual impairment, and any comorbidities are key to individualizing care and management plans for this diverse cohort [9, 15]. Administration of echocardiogram and electrocardiogram are essential to determining the state of cardiac function in these patients. Additional testing, such as exercise stress testing and supplemental imaging, may be indicated in specific patients [3, 9]. These assessments are important to properly gauge the propensity for these women to successfully cope with the physiologic demands of pregnancy, labor, and the peripartum period. In particular, the increased incidence of tachyarrhythmias coupled with the propensity to experience maladaptive cardiac pacemakers, chronotropic incompetence, and stenotic valves predispose these patients to decompensation during pregnancy [15].

Furthermore, when analyzing the medical histories of women with CHD, identifying their current medications is vital. Many diurnal medications that women with cardiac defects may take, like ACEs and ARBs, are generally avoided in pregnancy due to concern for adverse effects on fetal development [15]. Because these medications are often important to the management of cardiovascular pathology in this population, evaluating whether these patients may discontinue such therapies for extended periods of time during gestation is necessary. While providing preconception counseling to these women, it is worth considering short-term discontinuation of such medications to observe the effects on cardiac function and overall health of these patients prior to pregnancy [15].

Finally, subsequent to identifying the type of lesion and estimating the attributable morbidity and mortality in each patient, investigating opportunities for surgical or pharmacologic intervention is crucial. If an operative or pharmacologic remedy exists and the patient would tolerate pregnancy better if employed, then serious consideration should be given to undergoing treatment prior to pregnancy.

Table 2. Modified World Health Organization Pregnancy Risk Classification for Women with Congenital Heart Disease

WHO Pregnancy Risk Category	Risk Description	Specific Cardiac Lesions
I	No detectable increase in maternal mortality and no/ mild increase in morbidity risk	Uncomplicated small / mild pulmonary stenosis, patent ductus arteriosus, mitral valve prolapse
		Successfully repaired simple lesions: atrial septal defect, ventricular septal defect, patent ductus arteriosus, anomalous pulmonary venous drainage
		Isolated atrial or ventricular ectopic beats
II	Small increase in maternal mortality and moderate increase in morbidity risk	If otherwise well and uncomplicated:
		Unrepaired Atrial Septal Defect
		Repaired Tetralogy of Fallot
II-III	Moderate increase in maternal mortality & morbidity risk	Native or tissue valvular disease
		Aortic dilation 45 mm in bicuspid aortic valve aortopathy
		Repaired coarctation
		Tetralogy of Fallot
III	Significantly increased maternal mortality or severe morbidity risk. Expert counseling required. In the event of pregnancy, intensive specialist cardiac and obstetric monitoring needed throughout pregnancy, childbirth, and the puerperium.	Mechanical valve
		Systemic right ventricle
		Fontan circulation
		Cyanotic heart disease, unrepaired
		Aortic dilation
		Aortic dilation 45 - 50 mm in bicuspid aortic valve aortopathy
IV	Extremely high maternal mortality or severe morbidity risk pregnancy is contraindicated. In the event of pregnancy, termination should be discussed. In the event of pregnancy, intensive specialist cardiac and obstetric monitoring needed throughout pregnancy, childbirth, and the puerperium.	Pulmonary arterial hypertension
		Severe systemic ventricular dysfunction (LV ejection fraction < 30%)
		Severe aortic stenosis
		Severe mitral stenosis
		Eisenmenger syndrome
		Aortic dilation > 45 mm in Marfan syndrome
		Aortic dilation > 50 mm in aortic valve aortopathy
		Severe coarctation

ANTEPARTUM MANAGEMENT

Table 3. Multidisciplinary care and delivery plan checklist

History of congenital heart defect and current cardiovascular status: ☐ Formal diagnosis ☐ History of interventions and surgical procedures ☐ Residual cardiac lesions and current cardiovascular impairment ☐ Records of prior cardiovascular complications ☐ Current imaging of the anatomy of the patient's heart and any related arteriovenous anomalies

Current recommendations and considerations for baseline patient care and assessment
☐ Need for air-bubble filter for paradoxical embolism prophylaxis
    ☐ Yes
    ☐ No
☐ Alternative location for blood pressure monitoring due to prior surgical interventions preventing measurement in the upper extremities

☐ Expected complications :
☐ Type of complication
    ☐ Anticipated timing of complication
☐ Recommended interventions for potential complications including:
    ☐ Arrhythmia
    ☐ Heart failure
    ☐ Thromboembolus
    ☐ Other
☐ Contact information for members of the cardiology care team in event of complication
☐ Medications to be present and available on labor and delivery
    ☐ Indications for use of non-routine medications on labor and delivery
    ☐ Instructions for administration and dosing for non-routine medications

Guidelines for use of common medications administered in labor and delivery:
☐ Beta mimetics [terbutaline]
    ☐ No restrictions
    ☐ Use with caution
    ☐ Prohibited
☐ Misoprostol [cytotec]
    ☐ No restrictions
    ☐ Use with caution
    ☐ Prohibited
☐ Oxytocin
    ☐ No restrictions
    ☐ Use with caution
    ☐ Prohibited
☐ Prostaglandin F analogues [Carboprost/Hemabate]
    ☐ No restrictions
    ☐ Use with caution
    ☐ Prohibited
☐ Methergine
    ☐ No restrictions
    ☐ Use with caution
    ☐ Prohibited

❏	Comprehensive list of current medications
❏	Comprehensive list of allergies
❏	Past obstetric history
	❏ Delivery types
	❏ Complications
❏	Delivery Recommendations
	❏ Mode of delivery
	❏ Timing of delivery
	❏ Anesthesia considerations
	❏ Intrapartum cardiac monitoring
❏	Postpartum care
	❏ Location for postpartum care
	❏ ICU
	❏ Cardiology inpatient unit
	❏ General postpartum unit
	❏ Cardiac monitoring postpartum
	❏ Detailed postpartum care and assessment plans
	❏ Intake and output
	❏ Laboratory type and frequency
	❏ Consults
	❏ Postpartum imaging studies
❏	Follow up plans
	❏ Obstetrics
	❏ Cardiology
	❏ Other

The appropriate level of care should have been identified for women with CHD either prior to or early in pregnancy to ensure the necessary resources are available. Ideally women with complex CHD are cared for by a multidisciplinary team skilled and knowledgably in cardiac disease in pregnancy. Given the known increased risk of CHD in the offspring of pregnant women with CHD, a formal fetal echocardiogram between 18-22 weeks is indicated in all of these women. Consideration should be given for fetal growth assessment by ultrasound as women with CHD are at increased risk for fetal growth restriction.

A plan of care should be clearly outlined in the medical record of a pregnant woman with CHD including plan for delivery timing and route and postpartum considerations. (Table 3) Some women may not be candidates for vaginal delivery based on their specific lesions. If labor hasn't occurred spontaneously by 39-40 weeks consideration for induction of labor may be indicated in women with CHD. Some women at increased risk for arrhythmias may require cardiac monitoring in labor and postpartum. Also antibiotics for endocarditis prophylaxis should be considered in all women with CHD and given to those at increased risk of developing infective endocarditis [1, 14].

We will outline management recommendations for women with CHD in pregnancy by specific lesion type.

SEPTAL DEFECTS

Atrial Septal Defects

Atrial septal defects are among the most commonly encountered congenital cardiac lesion in pregnant women [10]. While most women with ASD tolerate pregnancy well, women with unrepaired ASD in pregnancy are prone to increased risk of arrhythmias, pre-eclampsia, intrauterine growth restriction, and fetal mortality [10, 15]. ASDs can remain asymptomatic and undiagnosed until the hemodynamic changes of pregnancy unveil their presence [16]. Over time, the left-to-right shunt can lead to right ventricular enlargement [10]. The increased fluid volume in pregnancy can further aggravate this problem. On chest x-ray, right atrial and ventricular enlargement, prominent pulmonary arteries, and plethoric lung fields may be observed.

Among the most prevalent complications of ASD in pregnancy are the development of arrhythmias secondary to right atrial enlargement [10]. ASD predisposes women to increased rates of atrial fibrillation and atrial flutter relative to the general population. Additionally, women 35 years and older who are diagnosed with large, uncorrected ASD are at increased risk of developing chronic atrial fibrillation, right ventricular dysfunction, and pulmonary hypertension [16]. Women who develop these complications should be cautioned against embarking on pregnancy.

In general, the standard management of arrhythmias with calcium channel blockers and beta-blockers is recommended. Patients who fail pharmacologic management and experience recurrent arrhythmias during pregnancy may be candidates for catheter ablation. Also consideration should be given for 0.22 micron filters on their IVs to avoid paradoxical bubble emboli when admitted for delivery.

Ventricular Septal Defects

Ventricular septal defects constitute the most prevalent congenital defect in the pregnant population. While VSDs limited to the muscular septum often resolve during childhood, defects present in the membranous segments of the ventricular septum commonly persist and can precipitate cardiopulmonary sequelae. Specifically, large patent VSDs can engender left ventricular overload and heart failure if left uncorrected. Similarly, chronic left-to-right shunting, increased pulmonary vascular resistance, and the development of Eisenmenger syndrome may develop in patients with large, unrepaired VSDs [10, 16]. Yet, despite the risks associated with large, complicated, and unrepaired VSD, small, simple, and repaired defects carry a good prognosis for pregnant patients and low likelihood of significant cardiac complications. Accordingly, large VSDs should ideally be surgically repaired before women become pregnant [10, 15]. Consideration should be given for 0.22 micron filters on their IVs to avoid paradoxical bubble emboli when admitted for delivery.

Patent Ductus Arteriosus

Patent ductus arteriosus is most often diagnosed in infancy. In pregnancy, PDA may be diagnosed on physical exam with classic machine-like holosystolic murmur. Chest x-ray may exhibit a slightly enlarged cardiac silhouette and EKG may exhibit left ventricular hypertrophy. If PDA was not repaired in infancy, occlusion of the PDA is encouraged prior to pregnancy via percutaneous intravascular catheter or open repair. Among patients who have a repaired PDA, uncomplicated PDA, and in whom left to right shunt is not associated with pulmonary hypertension, the pregnancy may progress safely without risk of significant complication. On the contrary, patients with unrepaired PDA with evidence of pulmonary hypertension are poor candidates for pregnancy and should be discouraged from becoming pregnant or offered termination if they are incidentally found to be pregnant at the time of presentation [16].

Eisenmenger Syndrome

Insofar as maternal and fetal morbidity and mortality are concerned, Eisenmenger syndrome is one of the most lethal conditions in pregnancy [3, 10, 16]. Eisenmenger syndrome is most often a complication of unrepaired ventricular septal defect or patent ductus arteriosus. Due to a maternal mortality rate of 30-50%, pregnancy is contraindicated in patients with Eisenmenger syndrome [3, 15, 16]. Equally grave, the risk of spontaneous pregnancy loss is also estimated to be nearly 50% among this subset of women [10]. Along with its lethality, Eisenmenger syndrome also portends higher incidences of intrauterine growth restriction and preterm labor [18]. Because of the degree of inherent risk, termination should be offered to these patients if they become pregnant. If they decide to continue with the pregnancy, close monitoring is imperative to monitor for signs of right sided heart failure [3, 10, 16]. These patients should be managed by a multidisciplinary team with expertise in complex cardiac disease in pregnancy and delivery should be at an advanced care center.

VALVULAR DEFECTS

Aortic Stenosis

Aortic stenosis is a common cause of left ventricular outflow obstruction and may be congenital or acquired. Among reproductive-aged women, congenital bicuspid valve is the most common cause of aortic stenosis [3, 10, 13, 16]. For many patients born with congenital aortic stenosis, the first time they will learn of their diagnosis is in adulthood. This is particularly true for women who may first become symptomatic in pregnancy [3, 10]. Other women may remain asymptomatic until they reach childbearing age. Therefore, a formal diagnosis and evaluation of any patient presenting with newly diagnosed or suspected aortic stenosis requires extensive diagnostic testing, detailed clinical history, and thorough physical exam.

Chief among the diagnostic testing available is echocardiography. Echocardiography allows the clinician to verify the diagnosis, examine the degree of stenosis, and identify any coexisting anomalies such as coarctation of the aorta and aortic dilatation [3, 13]. Because of the association of bicuspid aortic valves with aortopathies and aortic dilatation, additional imaging of the thoracic aorta is often necessary to quantify the degree of dilation of the aorta [3]. If the aortic diameter measurements exceed 50 mm, then surgical replacement of the ascending aorta is indicated prior to pregnancy [15].

Furthermore, in addition to performing echocardiography, patients with clinically silent aortic stenosis at time of presentation benefit greatly from undergoing exercise stress testing. Exercise stress testing allows the clinician to garner evidence of ischemic changes on EKGs, arrhythmias, diminished cardiac endurance, and abnormal hemodynamic responses when the heart is placed under significant stress as in pregnancy [3].

It is important to understand that there is a wide spectrum of disease among patients with aortic stenosis ranging from mild and asymptomatic to severe and debilitated. Consequently, the risks of adverse pregnancy outcomes varies as a direct function of disease severity. Asymptomatic patients diagnosed with mild to moderate aortic stenosis, for example, carry a low risk for complications and are generally expected to meet the demands of pregnancy well [3]. Normal exercise stress testing, adequate resting left ventricular function, and aortic valve peak pressures less than 80 mmHg are also good prognostic indicators that suggest patients will tolerate pregnancy well. Alternatively, symptomatic patients diagnosed with severe aortic stenosis and patients who fare poorly during exercise stress testing with signs of ventricular dysfunction, arrhythmia, and ineffective blood pressure accommodation are unlikely to be able to withstand the demands of pregnancy. These more vulnerable patients should be counseled against pregnancy [3]. Instead, patients with signs and symptoms of severe disease who desire to become pregnant should undergo valvuloplasty prior to pregnancy to decrease disease burden and improve prospective outcomes.

These patients are at high risk for adverse cardiac outcomes including the development of arrhythmias, angina, myocardial infarctions, and heart failure [3]. For those patients for whom the risk of complications secondary to the stress of labor is much greater a cesarean section should be considered [15]. Patients with severe aortic stenosis should be managed by a multidisciplinary team with expertise in complex cardiac disease in pregnancy and delivery should be at an advanced care center as valve replacement may be necessary during pregnancy or delivery.

Pulmonary Stenosis

Congenital pulmonic valve stenosis is a comparatively rare congenital defect most often seen in conjunction with other cardiac abnormalities [10]. Pulmonary stenosis occurs in approximately 5/10,000 live births and represents only 2% of CHD [10]. In general, most right ventricular outflow obstructions, including pulmonic stenosis, are at low risk for complications during pregnancy [3, 10, 15]. Yet, because patients with right ventricular outflow obstructions often have signs of right ventricular hypertrophy, the hypervolemic state of pregnancy may precipitate development of atrial arrhythmias and right sided heart failure [10, 15]. Similarly, the presence of significant pulmonic valve regurgitation must be considered in these patients and a detailed echocardiogram is important to evaluate the degree of valvular incompetence or stenosis. In patients with signs of severe pulmonic stenosis, defined by a peak-doppler-gradient in excess of 64 mmHg, intervention with intracatheter balloon valvuloplasty should be considered either pre-pregnancy or during pregnancy [3, 15]. Similarly, pulmonic valve replacement should be discussed in the setting of right ventricular dysfunction or symptomatic patients with signs of severe regurgitation.

While women with asymptomatic, uncomplicated pulmonary stenosis typically tolerate pregnancy well without concern for significant complications, there is evidence to suggest that, like many other patients with congenital cardiac lesions, an increased risk of pre-eclampsia and hypertensive disorders of pregnancy exists [15]. Likewise, elevated rates of miscarriage, preterm delivery, and inherited CHD in infants born to these women have been documented [13].

Owing to the low risk of complications in most women with pulmonic stenosis, vaginal delivery is recommended except in patients who are classified as NYHA class III/IV with evidence of severe pulmonic stenosis unresponsive to conservative management and ineligible for, or whom have failed, percutaneous valvular repair [15]. For those patients for whom the risk of complications secondary to the stress of labor is much greater a cesarean section should be considered [15]. Patients with severe pulmonary stenosis should be managed by a multidisciplinary team with expertise in complex cardiac disease in pregnancy and delivery should be at an advanced care center as valve replacement may be necessary during pregnancy or delivery.

COARCTATION OF THE AORTA

Nearly 6-8% of women born with CHD are found to have coarctation of the aorta CoA [2]. Approximately 80% of these women will be diagnosed in infancy or childhood [2]. While most women undergo surgical repair in childhood, some women may reach adulthood with undiagnosed coarctations [2]. Women with unrepaired or newly diagnosed CoA with significant hemodynamic symptoms should be counseled to undergo surgical correction before considering pregnancy.

Women with CoA are at risk for severe cardiovascular complications during pregnancy. Evidence suggests that 3-5% of pregnant women with CoA may be at risk for fatal complications [16]. In particular, CoA predisposes pregnant patients to intracranial hemorrhage secondary to increased risk of Berry aneurysms, elevated risk of chronic hypertension and hypertensive disorders of pregnancy, and aortic dilation and dissection [10, 15, 16].

Correspondingly, CoA is also correlated with increased rates of adverse neonatal outcomes [2, 3]. Specifically, higher rates of pregnancy loss, intrauterine growth restriction, placental abruption, and preterm delivery are more prevalent among women with CoA [2, 3, 15].

In general, many of the aforementioned complications are the result of longstanding poorly controlled hypertension resulting from CoA. Management of these patients, therefore, relies heavily upon effective blood pressure control with antihypertensives [2, 15, 16, 10]. However, employing antihypertensives in these patients risks inciting hypotension distal to the coarctation and resulting uterine hypoperfusion [10]. Patients with severe coarctation should similarly be managed by a multidisciplinary team with expertise in complex cardiac disease in pregnancy and delivery should be at an advanced care.

Ebstein's Anomaly

Ebstein's anomaly represents a rare congenital heart abnormality involving a malformed, downwardly displaced tricuspid valve that gives rise to an atrialized right ventricle and enlarged right atrium [11, 12]. It accounts for less than 1% of congenital heart defects [11, 12]. ASD and Wolf-Parkinson-White syndrome are frequently encountered in conjunction with the anomalous tricuspid valve [12, 15, 16]. Ebstein's anomaly generally carries a favorable prognosis for an overall uncomplicated pregnancy. It is especially important to evaluate the baseline functional status of these patients to accurately appraise their expected risks in pregnancy. Every patient with Ebstein's anomaly should undergo echocardiogram to assess the severity of their disease, anatomy, and cardiac function [12].

Patients with evidence of severe tricuspid regurgitation and heart failure are at increased risk for severe complications and should undergo treatment or be advised to avoid pregnancy [15] Moreover, evidence of worsening cardiopulmonary status, cyanosis, and underlying tricuspid regurgitation warrants recommending tricuspid valve replacement before contemplating pregnancy [12, 15, 16].

TETRALOGY OF FALLOT

Tetralogy of Fallot (ToF), the most common cyanotic heart defect, is defined by the presence of four cardiac malformations: a large VSD, an overriding aorta, severe pulmonary stenosis, and right ventricular hypertrophy [17]. ToF exists along a continuum with varying degrees of severity related to the extent of right ventricular outflow obstruction and the size of the septal defect [16]. ToF is also associated with 22q11 chromosomal deletions in 15% of patients and 5-10% of infants born to women with ToF are at risk of inheritance. It is therefore important to offer women contemplating pregnancy genetic counseling to discuss the risks of inheritance in their offspring. While the majority of patients in industrialized nations undergo surgical intervention early in life to repair the septal defect and alleviate the stenosis of the pulmonary valve by enlarging the ventricular infundibulum, women born in developing countries with limited access to advanced healthcare may present with unrepaired ToF lesions [16, 18].

Overall, women with asymptomatic, post-repair ToF without evidence of pulmonary regurgitation, right ventricular dysfunction, or obstruction typically have favorable pregnancy outcomes [16]. On the contrary, data suggests that women with unrepaired ToF may carry a 15% risk of maternal mortality and 30% risk of fetal loss during pregnancy [18]. Due to the profound maternal and fetal mortality associated with unrepaired ToF, surgical repair is indicated before considering childbearing. Patients with unrepaired ToF should be cautioned to delay or avoid pregnancy until palliative surgery has been performed and further evaluation of cardiac function is completed. Surgical repair, however, is not curative [16]. Even among women with repaired ToF cardiac, complications can occur in over 10% of patients [15]. Arrhythmias and heart failure represent the two most common complications while thromboembolism, aortic root dilation, and endocarditis are also frequently seen. Furthermore, pregnancy should also be discouraged in patients with evidence of hematocrit greater than 60%, right ventricular systolic pressure greater than 120 mmHg, and a history of multiple syncopal episodes as they are at considerable risk for severe complications and poor outcomes.

Of similar concern among this population are women presenting with signs of cyanosis. Cyanotic patients represent another sub-group of patients with ToF who carry a poor prognosis and elevated risk for adverse outcomes. The decreased systemic vascular resistance characteristic of pregnancy can exacerbate the left-to-right shunt present in patients with ToF. Increased shunting can potentiate hypoxemia resulting in syncope and death [16]. These risks are greatest during the third trimester and in the immediate postpartum period. Special attention should be paid to ensure adequate venous return is maintained. Patients should be informed of these risks and counseled to wear compression stockings during late pregnancy [15, 16].

During pregnancy, patients who have undergone reparative surgery and who are asymptomatic may safely be monitored each trimester by their cardiologist. Conversely, patients with evidence of hematocrit greater than 60%, right ventricular systolic pressure greater than 120 mmHg, and a history of multiple syncopal episodes are at considerable risk for severe complications and poor outcomes and necessitate closer monitoring [3]. Patients with evidence of pulmonary regurgitation are also at elevated risk and should be evaluated with echocardiography on a monthly basis to assess cardiac function as the pregnancy progresses [15]. In patients who experience continued deterioration of cardiac function leading to right ventricular failure, diuretics and bed-rest are recommended [15]. If conservative management with diuretics and bed-rest fails, however, it is recommended that transcatheter valve implantation be considered [15].

Typically, women born with ToF today undergo surgical repair enabling them to enjoy generally safe and low risk pregnancies [3, 15]. Nevertheless, given the variety of clinical features embodied by the spectrum of disease among patients born with ToF, and the unique clinical histories of each patient, it is crucial to tailor care and counseling to the specific needs of each individual to ensure the best and safest outcomes for every mother and child.

TRANSPOSITION OF THE GREAT VESSELS

Transposition of the great vessels represents two congenital malformations: D-transposition of the great arteries [D-TGA] and L-transposition of the great arteries or congenitally corrected transposition of the great arteries [CC-TGA] [3]. The important distinction between these two abnormalities relies on the presence of ventricular inversion, in addition to inversion of the great arteries, in the setting of CC-TGA [3]. Ventricular inversion enables normal physiologic circulation whereby the right ventricle acts as the systemic pump and may or may not require surgical correction depending on the co-existing structural abnormalities. Conversely, D-TGA is incompatible with survival and requires surgical repair [3]. Most commonly, the Senning or Mustard atrial switch procedures have been performed to remedy circulation abnormalities and prevent the development of cyanosis and long-term sequelae [3, 15, 16]. Although the arterial switch procedure corrects circulation abnormalities, the right ventricle remains in the systemic position lending to a myriad of adverse effects [3, 16].

Both patients with D-TGA status post arterial switch and CC-TGA are vulnerable to the physiologic changes and demands of pregnancy. Data from one large multicenter trial demonstrated a 36% risk for cardiac complications during the third trimester in these patients [10]. Complications typically include worsening or new arrhythmias, especially along atrial suture lines, heart failure, and exacerbation of pre-existing tricuspid regurgitation [3, 10].

Given the high likelihood of poor outcomes among these patients, determining the patient's functional status is integral to risk stratification and proper pre-conception and pregnancy planning. Completion of an EKG, echocardiogram or MRI, exercise stress testing, and Holter monitoring are fundamental tests to adequately assess valvular and ventricular function [2]. Counseling patients categorized as NYHA Class III/IV [or WHO Class III/IV] due to impaired ventricular function against pregnancy is warranted [3, 15].

Those patients who go on to become pregnant merit a repeat EKG and echocardiogram [3, 15]. Should ventricular dysfunction be suspected a BNP may be ordered [15]. This may serve as a benchmark of ventricular function as the patient progresses through pregnancy. Going forward, patients are recommended to undergo close surveillance by their cardiologists every 4-6 weeks through the second trimester and every 2-4 weeks during the third trimester [15]. Detailed delivery plans and instructions should be composed by the multidisciplinary care team [3, 15]. Vaginal delivery is indicated with facilitated second stage of labor and administration regional anesthesia. Cesarean delivery is not indicated for cardiovascular reasons and should therefore be reserved for obstetric concerns [3, 15]. Moreover, in addition to cardiac complications in the mother, patients with TGA are at increased risk for pre-eclampsia and fetal complications relative to uncomplicated pregnancies [10].

Lastly, during the immediate postpartum period patients with TGA are at elevated risk for exacerbated or new onset heart failure and arrhythmias [3, 10, 16]. Cardiac monitoring and close nursing supervision is thus critical to evaluate for signs and symptoms of volume overload or arrhythmias in the first 24-48 hours postpartum [3]. For the remainder of puerperium patients should be closely monitored to identify signs of cardiovascular decompensation as worsening functional status is common in from 3-5 days postpartum through 6 months after delivery [3].

FONTAN CIRCULATION IN WOMEN WITH UNIVENTRICULAR HEARTS AND SINGLE-VENTRICLE PHYSIOLOGY

Until recently, women born with single-ventricle physiology and univentricular cardiac anomalies had a poor overall prognosis. With the development of the Fontan procedure, however, the 10 year survival rate is now approximately 85% [18]. The Fontan procedure represents a palliative surgical intervention originally employed to mitigate the effects of tricuspid atresia, but now performed to alleviate many of the complications resulting from a variety of conditions defined by single-ventricle physiology cardiac anomalies [3, 10]. In essence, the Fontan procedure redirects systemic circulation directly into the pulmonary artery, thereby bypassing the right heart and single ventricle or intervening cardiac pump [10, 18].

Although the procedure remedies the cyanosis associated with these conditions, it is also responsible for an array of complications that present longstanding challenges to the health and wellbeing of these patients [3]. This is especially true when under the duress of the cardiac demands and hemodynamic changes in pregnancy.

Specifically, chronic elevation of systemic venous pressure, decreased cardiac output, and decreased cardiac reserve ensue after the procedure. Over time, the patient becomes susceptible to the development of edema, ascites, cardiac insults, and atrial arrhythmias secondary to diminished ventricular function, protein-loss enteropathy, portal hypertension, and thromboembolic events [3, 10, 18].

Despite the potential for well tolerated pregnancies, these patients are still at an overwhelmingly high risk for severe maternal and fetal adverse outcomes. Upwards of 2% of women with Fontan circulation, even those who may be candidates for pregnancy, remain at risk for fatal complications and death [18]. Fetal and obstetric complications are also much more prevalent among these patients. Increased rates of miscarriage, fetal demise, preterm delivery, premature rupture of membranes, and IUGR have been reported [3].

Thus, due to the overwhelmingly high levels of severe morbidity and mortality incurred by these patients termination is offered. If pregnancy continues we recommend close monitoring throughout pregnancy and postpartum is recommended. Immediately after pregnancy is confirmed, care should be established with a multidisciplinary care team with experience and expertise in treating patients with Fontan circulation [3, 15]. Care should be transferred to a tertiary care center equipped to manage these patients effectively. A timely and comprehensive physical exam, obstetric history, and inventory of all cardiac medications must be performed. Baseline testing should include liver function tests and arterial oxygen saturation measurements. During each subsequent clinic visit providers should ensure that oxygen saturation is measured and trended throughout the pregnancy. Serial echocardiograms should be completed each trimester to continuously monitor ventricular function as these patients are at heightened risk for decompensation [15]. Likewise, Holter monitoring should be considered in patients presenting with complaints of palpitations or histories of arrhythmias [3, 15].

Because patients with Fontan circulation are at increased risk of thromboembolism, anticoagulation with LMWH is indicated in women with evidence of a prior embolic event or women with diagnosis of atrial arrhythmias [3].

While women who remain asymptomatic may be permitted to continue with their routine activities, they should be counseled that they are at increased risk for deteriorating functional status as pregnancy proceeds. Patients should be educated to monitor sodium intake, take reats, and refrain from excessive strenuous exercise [3, 15, 16]. Likewise, patients should be informed of the importance of reporting any signs or symptoms of decreased capacity such as unresolving palpitations, peripheral edema, and dyspnea [3, 16].

Delivery is indicated in symptomatic patients at 37-38 weeks or earlier as clinically indicated [3, 15]. All women admitted to L&D with a history of Fontan circulation should receive cardiac monitoring, compression stockings, IV access, and pulse oximetry monitoring [3]. If the risk of air emboli is elevated due to the presence of shunts found in the patient, IV air filters should be considered [3].

Vaginal delivery is acceptable for women with Fontan circulation in most circumstances. Women should be encouraged to labor in the left lateral position to maximize venous return [3, 16]. In order to shorten the duration of the second stage, an assisted second stage is recommended with the use of regional anesthesia [3, 10]. In patients with evidence of heart failure or arrhythmia an early delivery or cesarean section may be indicated [3, 15]. Should patients show signs of decompensation such as hypoxia, interventions such as supplemental oxygen and arterial line placement are prudent. Patients who are stable after delivery may be admitted to the general postpartum unit with 24 hours of cardiac monitoring and close nursing supervision. For unstable patients with signs of impaired cardiac function, admission to the intensive care unit is recommended [3]. Continued close surveillance of these patients should extend through 4-6 weeks postpartum as they remain at risk for severe complications throughout the puerperium [3].

POSTPARTUM CARE AND MANAGEMENT

Soon after delivery, significant alterations to maternal physiology, once again, occur. Most notably, the involution of the uterus yields a 500 mL auto-transfusion within the maternal circulation that magnifies maternal intravascular volume. At the same time, maternal cardiac activity is augmented to contend with the significant hemodynamic changes underway. Namely, increases in stroke volume and cardiac output develop. In healthy patients, wiithout history of cardiovascular disease, stroke volume may increase upwards 71% whereas cardiac output may rise by 60-80%. In general, the changes seen in the immediate postpartum period largely revert to baseline during the first 48 hours postpartum. While a full resolution of hemodynamic changes is often observed during the first 6-8 weeks postpartum, some effects can last for nearly half a year [3, 18].

Although most women contend with these significant physiologic changes well, they present a substantial challenge to women with preexisting cardiopulmonary disease with impaired cardiovascular function. Given that many of these hemodynamic changes occur simultaneously in the early postpartum period, contending with them concurrently may overwhelm the cardiovascular systems of women with CHD. Burdening these already strained cardiovascular systems can lead to complications and decompensation postpartum. It is therefore especially important to recognize women who would benefit from increased levels of postpartum care and monitoring to effectively monitor, manage, and respond to such events.

For example, patients with arrhythmias diagnosed antepartum or intrapartum demand heightened surveillance after delivery. Telemetry services should be employed for the first 24-48 hours postpartum in patients with elevated risk of arrhythmia. Additionally, women who exhibit signs or symptoms of heart failure, cardiopulmonary decompensation, or who are at elevated risk for decompensation secondary to their respective underlying anomalies, require increased levels of care not routinely available in general postpartum wards. For such patients, admission to an intensive care unit for the initial 24-48 hours postpartum is advisable. Transfer to an ICU may allow such patients to access both cardiac monitoring and specialized staff with expertise in the management of cardiac critical care. Procuring placement in an ICU is thus instrumental to early identification and intervention of cardiopulmonary decompensation among postpartum patients with CHD [3].

Conversely, admission to a general postpartum unit is reasonable for patients with CHD who remained stable and withstood the burden of gestation without significant complications. Nevertheless, nursing and ancillary staff in general postpartum units caring for such patients should be educated on clinical signs and symptoms for which to monitor to prevent significant decompensation or adverse events. Likewise, routine care of postpartum patients with CHD should include early ambulation and continued use of sequential compression devices and support stockings to decrease risk of thromboembolism [3].

Lastly, contraception should be a routine topic of discussion broached with all patients during pregnancy. Among women with CHD, contraceptive counseling should be an ongoing discussion throughout their reproductive lives and childbearing years. While preconception counseling on contraception is optimal, recurrent discussions about contraceptive options with pregnant patients, especially those with CHD, is necessary and should be a routine aspect of postpartum care.

Contraceptive counseling should take into account the patient's desires for future fertility, the risks associated with unplanned pregnancies, contraindications to contraceptives relative to the patient's unique medical history and current state of health, and anticipated compliance with potential contraceptive regimens. Depending on each of these factors, specific classes of contraceptives may be more or less idea for each individual patient [3].

Combined contraceptive options that contain both estrogen and progesterone are desirable for patients interested in predictable menstrual cycles. In addition, combined options are highly effective and may reduce the risk of gynecologic cancers later in life. Yet, estrogen-containing contraception poses an increased risk of thromboembolism [3]. Owing to the hypercoagulable state during pregnancy and into the early postpartum period, estrogens containing contraceptive methods are generally avoided for the first several weeks postpartum [3]. Patients with a history of a thrombus should not be offered estrogen containing contraceptive methods given this increased risk [5, 3]. Likewise, patients with a history of myocardial infarction, ischemic heart disease, stroke, inherited hypercoagulable disorders, migraine with aura, pulmonary hypertension, poorly controlled severe hypertension, and concurrent significant tobacco use over the age of 35 [>15 cigarettes per day] should all be counseled against the use of estrogen containing contraceptives as well [5]. While this list is not exhaustive, it demonstrates the detailed counseling necessary to properly advise patients on the most safe and appropriate contraceptive method for them.

Apart from combined estrogen-progesterone options, progesterone only options like the progesterone-only pill, medroxyprogesterone acetate injections [depo-provera injections], subdermal implants,and levonorgestrel intrauterine devices] provide alternative options for patients for whom estrogen may be an absolute or relative contraindication [3]. As for non-hormonal intrauterine devices such as the copper-basedIUD, the aforementioned levonorgestrel IUD is considered preferable due to risks of heavy menstrual bleeding and resulting anemia that may pose undue strain on patients with CHD [3].

Moreover, if patients have completed their childbearing, and are interested in permanent sterilization options, bilateral tubal ligation procedures should be discussed and offered [3]. These methods may provide effective long-term contraception for women who no longer plan to get pregnant or for whom future pregnancy is contraindicated due to associated risks.

CONCLUSION

Advancements in medical, surgical, and diagnostic techniques continue to improve the livelihoods of patients born with congenital heart defects. The growing cohort of reproductive aged women born with CHD necessitates specialized care tailored to this unique patient population. While the evidence suggests that many, perhaps even the majority, of these women may enjoy normal, uncomplicated pregnancies and deliveries, the risk for severe complications and poor outcomes remains an important consideration. It is therefore the responsibility of clinicians to develop a comprehensive multi-disciplinary approach to individualize care and management of these patients. Working together, clinicians across specialties can share their expertise to provide these patients with effective counseling, planning, and management of their pregnancies to promote successful and safe outcomes.

REFERENCES

[1] "ACOG Practice Bulletin No. 199 Summary." *Obstetrics & Gynecology* 132, no. 3 [2018]: 798-800. doi:10.1097/aog.0000000000002834.

[2] Beauchesne, Luc M, Heidi M Connolly, Naser M Ammash, and Carole A Warnes. "Coarctation of the Aorta: Outcome of Pregnancy." *Journal of the American College of Cardiology* 38, no. 6 [2001]: 1728–33. https://doi.org/10.1016/s0735-1097[01]01617-5.

[3] Canobbio, Mary M., Carole A. Warnes, Jamil Aboulhosn, Heidi M. Connolly, Amber Khanna, Brian J. Koos, Seema Mital, Carl Rose, Candice Silversides, and Karen Stout. "Management of Pregnancy in Patients With Complex Congenital Heart Disease: A Scientific Statement for Healthcare Professionals From the American Heart Association." *Circulation* 135, no. 8 [2017]. https://doi.org/10.1161/cir.0000000000000458.

[4] "Cardiovascular Physiology of Pregnancy." Circulation. https://ww w.ahajournals.org/doi/full/10.1161/circulationaha.114.009029.

[5] "CDC - Summary Chart: Hormonal Contraceptive Methods and IUDs - USMEC - Reproductive Health." Centers for Disease Control and Prevention. Centers for Disease Control and Prevention. Accessed June 19, 2019. https://www.cdc.gov/reproductivehealth/contracepti on/mmwr/mec/appendixk.html#mec_cardio.

[6] Elkayam, Uri, Sorel Goland, Petronella G. Pieper, and Candice K. Silversides. "High-Risk Cardiac Disease in Pregnancy." *Journal of the American College of Cardiology*68, no. 5 [2016]: 502-16. doi:10.1 016/j.jacc.2016.05.050.

[7] Garbi, Madalina, and Chris Allen. "Faculty of 1000 Evaluation for 2017 AHA/ACC Focused Update of the 2014 AHA/ACC Guideline for the Management of Patients with Valvular Heart Disease: A Report of the American College of Cardiology/american Heart Association Task Force on Clinical Practice Guidelines." *F1000 - Post-publication Peer Review of the Biomedical Literature*, 2017. doi:10.3410/f.72742 6955.793533368.

[8] Gilboa, Suzanne M., Owen J. Devine, James E. Kucik, Matthew E. Oster, Tiffany Riehle-Colarusso, Wendy N. Nembhard, Ping Xu, Adolfo Correa, Kathy Jenkins, and Ariane J. Marelli. "Congenital Heart Defects in the United States." *Circulation*134, no. 2 [December 2016]: 101–9. https://doi.org/10.1161/circulationaha.115.019307.

[9] Greutmann, Matthias, and Petronella G. Pieper. "Pregnancy in Women with Congenital Heart Disease." *European Heart Journal*36, no. 37 [2015]: 2491–99. https://doi.org/10.1093/eurheartj/ehv288.

[10] Harris, Ian S. "Management of Pregnancy in Patients with Congenital Heart Disease." *Progress in Cardiovascular Diseases*53, no. 4 [2011]: 305–11. https://doi.org/10.1016/j.pcad.2010.08.001.

[11] Jost, Christine H. Attenhofer, Heidi M. Connolly, Joseph A. Dearani, William D. Edwards, and Gordon K. Danielson. "Ebstein's Anomaly." *Circulation*115, no. 2 [2007]: 277–85. https://doi.org/10.1161/circu lationaha.106.619338.

[12] Katsuragi, Shinji, Chizuko Kamiya, Kaoru Yamanaka, Reiko Neki, Takekazu Miyoshi, Naoko Iwanaga, Chinami Horiuchi, et al. "Risk Factors for Maternal and Fetal Outcome in Pregnancy Complicated by Ebstein Anomaly." *American Journal of Obstetrics and Gynecology* 209, no. 5 [2013]. https://doi.org/10.1016/j.ajog.2013.07.005.

[13] Lindley, Kathryn, and Dominique Williams. "Valvular Heart Disease in Pregnancy." American College of Cardiology, February 12, 2018. https://www.acc.org/latest-in-cardiology/articles/2018/02/12/07/29/valvular-heart-disease-in-pregnancy.

[14] Nishimura, Rick A., Catherine M. Otto, Robert O. Bonow, Blase A. Carabello, John P. Erwin, Lee A. Fleisher, Hani Jneid, Michael J. Mack, Christopher J. Mcleod, Patrick T. O'Gara, Vera H. Rigolin, Thoralf M. Sundt, and Annemarie Thompson. "2017 AHA/ACC Focused Update of the 2014 AHA/ACC Guideline for the Management of Patients With Valvular Heart Disease." *Journal of the American College of Cardiology* 70, no. 2 [2017]: 252-89. doi:10.1016/j.jacc.2017.03.011.

[15] Regitz-Zagrosek, V., Blomstrom Lundqvist, C., Borghi, C., Cifkova, R., Ferreira, R., Foidart, J., Gibbs, J., Gohlke-Baerwolf, C., Gorenek, B., Iung, B., Kirby, M., Maas, A., Morais, J., Nihoyannopoulos, P., Pieper, P., Presbitero, P., Roos-Hesselink, J., Schaufelberger, M., Seeland, U., Torracca, L., Bax, J., Auricchio, A., Baumgartner, H., Ceconi, C., Dean, V., Deaton, C., Fagard, R., Funck-Brentano, C., Hasdai, D., Hoes, A., Knuuti, J., Kolh, P., McDonagh, T., Moulin, C., Poldermans, D., Popescu, B., Reiner, Z., Sechtem, U., Sirnes, P., Torbicki, A., Vahanian, A., Windecker, S., Baumgartner, H., Deaton, C., Aguiar, C., Al-Attar, N., Garcia, A., Antoniou, A., Coman, I., Elkayam, U., Gomez-Sanchez, M., Gotcheva, N., Hilfiker-Kleiner, D., Kiss, R., Kitsiou, A., Konings, K., Lip, G., Manolis, A., Mebaaza, A., Mintale, I., Morice, M., Mulder, B., Pasquet, A., Price, S., Priori, S., Salvador, M., Shotan, A., Silversides, C., Skouby, S., Stein, J., Tornos, P., Vejlstrup, N., Walker, F. and Warnes, C. [2011]. ESC Guidelines on the management of cardiovascular diseases during pregnancy: The

Task Force on the Management of Cardiovascular Diseases during Pregnancy of the European Society of Cardiology [ESC]. *European Heart Journal*, 32[24], pp.3147-3197.

[16] Resnik, Robert. *Creasy and Resniks Maternal-Fetal Medicine: Principles and Practice*. Elsevier, 2019.

[17] Schlichting, Lauren E., Tabassum Z. Insaf, Ali N. Zaidi, George K. Lui, and Alissa R. Van Zutphen. "Maternal Comorbidities and Complications of Delivery in Pregnant Women with Congenital Heart Disease." *Journal of the American College of Cardiology* 73, no. 17 [2019]: 2181–91. https://doi.org/10.1016/j.jacc.2019.01.069.

[18] Simpson, Lynn L. "Maternal Cardiac Disease." *Obstetrics & Gynecology* 119, no. 2, Part 1 [2012]: 345–59. https://doi.org/10.1097/aog.0b013e318242e260.

In: Congenital Heart Disease
Editor: Curtis Giguère

ISBN: 978-1-53616-674-3
© 2020 Nova Science Publishers, Inc.

Chapter 3

CARDIAC RESYNCHRONIZATION THERAPY IN ADULTS WITH CONGENITAL HEART DISEASE: CURRENT STATE AND FUTURE PERSPECTIVES

Rohit K. Kharbanda[1,2], Ad J. J. C. Bogers[2] and Natasja M. S. de Groot[1],*

[1]Department of Cardiology, Erasmus Medical Center, Rotterdam, the Netherlands
[2]Department of Cardiothoracic Surgery, Erasmus Medical Center, Rotterdam, the Netherlands

ABSTRACT

Advances in therapy have resulted in an ever-increasing population of grown-ups with congenital heart disease (GUCH), also called adults with congenital heart disease (CHD), in whom sudden cardiac death and progressive heart failure are predominant causes of mortality. Treatment of

---

* Corresponding Author's Email: n.m.s.degroot@erasmusmc.nl.

adults with CHD in the setting of heart failure is challenging due to heterogeneity of the underlying anatomy and physiology, surgical scars, residual shunts and valvular dysfunction. Since donor hearts are scarce, worldwide interest has increased to apply cardiac resynchronization therapy (CRT) in this relatively young population. CRT is an established therapy for heart failure in patients with idiopathic or ischemic heart disease and electromechanical dyssynchronous ventricles. European and American guidelines provide specific indications for CRT in these patient groups, however these criteria are not directly applicable to patients with CHD. Since there are no randomized controlled trials in patients with CHD, the recommendations for CRT in this patient population is extrapolated from relatively small retrospective studies. Results from current retrospective studies are promising, however there are some major limitations. Relatively small number of patients in a heterogeneous group (including both pediatrics and adults) and a limited follow-up duration are important shortcomings of these studies, precluding long term outcomes. Moreover, patients with cardiomyopathies and congenital atrioventricular block are often included as patients with 'CHD' leading to results representing the outcome in a mixed population. The current GUCH guidelines do not provide indications for CRT as evidence supporting CRT has thus far been limited to case reports and retrospective studies in a heterogeneous patient population with different underlying cardiac defects. For the challenging systemic RV population, the guidelines state that CRT is still experimental. In these patients, the benefits of CRT are less clear. In the following chapter, current experience of CRT in adults with CHD is summarized and future perspectives are discussed.

Keywords: cardiac resynchronization therapy, congenital heart disease, heart failure

INTRODUCTION

With a reported incidence and prevalence of respectively 10 per 1000 and 3-20 per 1000 live births, congenital heart disease is the most common congenital anomaly diagnosed in newborns with major impact on public health (Tennant et al. 2010, van der Bom et al. 2011). Advances in therapy over the past decades have resulted in an ever-increasing population of grown-ups with congenital heart disease (GUCH), also called adults with congenital heart disease (CHD), in whom progressive heart failure and sudden cardiac death (SCD) are predominant causes of mortality (Marelli et al. 2014, Nieminen, Jokinen, and Sairanen 2007, Oechslin et al. 2000, Zomer et al. 2013). Improvement in life expectancy goes hand in hand with increased risk of (fatal) tachyarrhythmias and heart failure. The GUCH population contains patients with different underlying defects, different history of surgical procedures and subsequent different cardiac anatomy/physiology. Subsequently, the pathophysiology of heart failure in adults with CHD is divers, complex and multifactorial. Moreover, clinical presentation of these patients with heart failure differs per (residual) defect and age.

Adults with CHD is a challenging patient group for clinicians as current guideline recommendations are often based on expert opinions, case series and retrospective studies in heterogeneous study populations with different underling cardiac defects (Ponikowski et al. 2016, Yancy et al. 2017). This has resulted in a worldwide interest in adults with CHD regarding heart failure treatment. Since donor hearts are scarce, a worldwide interest in alternative treatment modalities such as cardiac resynchronization therapy (CRT) has increased. CRT is an established therapy for heart failure patients with idiopathic or ischemic heart disease and electromechanical dyssynchronous ventricles. Retrospective studies of CRT therapy in CHD patients are promising, however limited by the mixed populations (adults and pediatrics patients with different CHD) and the aforementioned limitations. Importantly, these studies are also limited by the follow-up duration, thereby precluding long-term outcomes and mortality rates (Dubin et al. 2005, Janousek et al. 2009, Cecchin et al. 2009). In this chapter, we discuss the current state and future perspectives of CRT in adults with CHD.

BASIC PRINCIPLES OF CARDIAC RESYNCHRONIZATION THERAPY

In the normal heart, atrial activation originates from the sinus node and propagates through both atria to reach the atrioventricular node. The electrical impulse is then conducted through the bundle of His, to the right and left bundle branch (existing of the anterior and posterior left bundle branch). Subsequently, the purkinje network activates the ventricles and ventricular contraction is initiated. The interaction between coordinated electrical activation of both ventricles and subsequent contraction is important for synchronous and hence efficient ventricular contraction. Dysfunction of the conduction system, which is often the case in patients with CHD, leads to electrical conduction through myocardial tissue. This results in slow, asynchronous electrical conduction and thus also asynchronous mechanical contraction of the ventricles. On the long-term a vicious circle is gradually formed, in which inefficient activation and contraction of the ventricles leads to decline in ventricular function, and eventually detrimental ventricular remodeling.

Application of CRT synchronizes electrical activation and mechanical contraction of both ventricles. This results in improvement of ventricular function and reverses ventricular remodeling resulting in improved quality of life and eventually lower mortality rates.

Current State of Cardiac Resynchronization Therapy for the Failing Systemic Left Ventricle

Cardiac resynchronization therapy (CRT) was introduced in the early 1990s as a novel therapy for heart failure. Outcomes of novel drugs were disappointing and electrical therapy gained interest. Observational studies demonstrated a positive effect of CRT in the treatment of heart failure.

Subsequently, large randomized controlled trials on CRT in patients with ischemic or idiopathic heart failure demonstrated a significant reduction in New York Heart Association (NYHA) class, increase in ventricular function, less hospitalization rates and decrease in use of heart failure medication (Abraham et al. 2002, Moss et al. 2009). Moreover, CRT implementation in relatively asymptomatic patients with low ejection fraction and prolonged QRS duration resulted in a lower risk of future heart-failure events. Patients included in large randomized trials investigating the outcome of CRT in ischemic heart disease are typical heart failure patients with left ventricular ejection fraction ≤30%, left bundle branch block and NYHA class III/IV. However, adults with CHD often have a right bundle branch block with complex anatomy and different physiologic conditions and are therefore not comparable with heart failure patients in whom ischemic heart disease is the principal etiology of heart failure. Hence, the efficacy of CRT in adults with CHD has not been established yet.

The first single center retrospective study, published by Strieper et al. in 2004, describes the initial experience of CRT in 6 pediatric and one adult patient (age 7 [2-28] years) with CHD. After a median follow-up period of 19 months, 5 patients, including the adult patient, had improved ejection fraction and reduction of symptoms. Thus, short term results seemed promising, though the study population was small and heterogeneous.

The second study was a multicenter study including 103 patients (age 13 [0-55] years) (Dubin et al. 2005). The main objective of this study was to examine CRT outcomes in pediatrics with CHD. Thirty out of 103 patients had a cardiomyopathy or a congenital heart block resulting in 73 (71%) patients with CHD. Despite their main objective to examine the outcome in pediatrics, 21 patients were older than 20 years and 23 patients were between 15-20 years of age.

Not only patients with systemic left ventricles, but also patients with systemic right ventricles (n = 17) and Fontan patients (n = 7) were included. After a median follow-up duration of 4 [0-12] months, mean QRS duration decreased by 37.7 ± 30.7ms, ejection fraction increased by 12.8 ± 12.7% and 11 patients were identified as non-responders (11%). Again, initial results were promising, yet the patient population was heterogeneous in addition to a limited follow-up duration.

The second retrospective multicenter study was published in 2009 by Janoušek et al. and included 109 patients (age: 17 [3-74] years) (Janoušek 2009). Eighty-seven (80%) patients had CHD and a mix of systemic right/left and Fontan patients were included. After a median follow-up duration of 7.5 months there was improvement in left ventricular ejection fraction and a decrease in QRS duration. This is the first study performing multivariate analyses on risk factors for non-responders, resulting in identification of poor initial NYHA class (≥III) as an independent predictor of non-response. However, other most likely important variables were not tested, such as age at CRT, differences between systemic right or left ventricle, ventricular pacing prior to CRT and lead position.

Recent reports by the German National Register for Congenital Heart Defects on CRT in CHD patients (n = 65, age 21.5 [8.7-37.7] years) with a follow-up duration of 7 years showed similar promising outcomes (Flügge et al. 2018).

So far, all prior studies reported on outcomes in both pediatric and adult patients with CHD. The first study investigating the efficacy of CRT in adults only was published in 2018 (Koyak et al. 2018). A total of 48 adults (47 [18-74] years) with a follow-up duration of 2.6 [0.1-8.8] years were retrospectively analyzed. Overall, 77% (n = 37) responded to CRT either by improvement in NYHA class or in systemic ventricular function. Three out of 11 non-responders died and four underwent a heart transplantation. This study demonstrates that CRT in adults with CHD is effective in the majority of the patients, however the small sample sized impeded risk factor analyses.

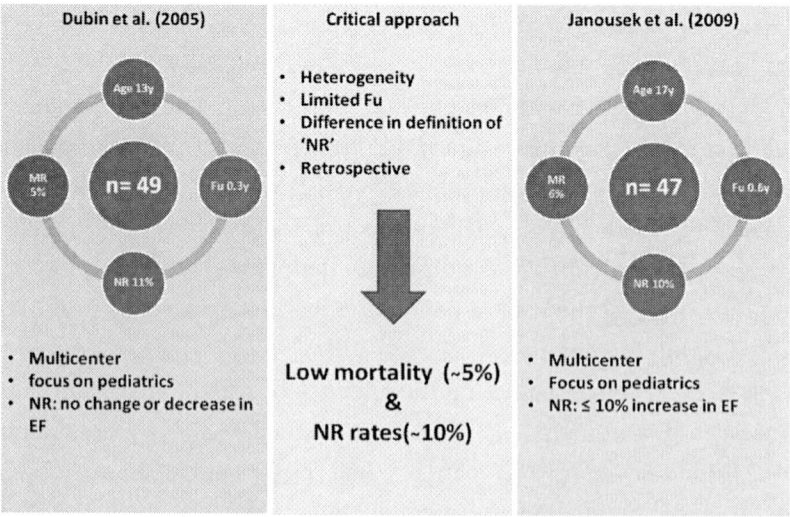

F = Ejection fraction, Fu = Follow-up, MR = Mortality, NR = Non-responder.

Figure 1. Two multicenter studies on outcome of CRT in adults with CHD.

Current evidence, which is based on retrospective studies, suggests that CRT is an important adjunctive therapy for adults with CHD and heart failure. The two largest multicenter studies are summarized in Figure 1. Future multicenter studies are essential to overcome limitations of current studies on CRT in patients with CHD and provide more robust evidence for both adults and pediatrics separately.

CARDIAC RESYNCHRONIZATION THERAPY FOR THE FAILING SYTEMIC RIGHT VENTRICLE

The first study reporting on outcomes of CRT in patients with CHD included only patients with a systemic right ventricle (Janoušek et al. 2004). Eight patients (age 13 [7-29] years), including three adults, with a systemic right ventricle (congenitally corrected transposition of the great arteries (cc-TGA)) were retrospectively analyzed in order to examine the acute and mid-term effects of CRT in this specific population. After a median follow-up duration of 17.4 [7.7-19.7] months, a significant decrease in QRS duration and increase in systemic right ventricular function was observed. This proof of concept study demonstrated that CRT may be promising in "preventing" progression of right ventricular failure in this high-risk population.

The two multicenter studies described above, also included patients with a systemic right ventricle (Dubin et al. 2005, Janoušek 2009). Dubin et al. included 17 patients (age: 12.7 [4.9-50] years, not specified how many adults) with TGA and observed a non-responder rate of 23.5% (Dubin et al. 2005). In the other multicenter study, 27 patients (median age: 28.8y) with a systemic right ventricle were included (Janoušek 2009) and only 13.6% of these patients were non-responders.

The former study defined non-responder as either no change or deterioration in systemic ventricular function. However, in the latter study, non-responders were defined as not only no improvement in systemic ventricular function but also no clinical response defined as a decrease in

NYHA class. Worldwide consensus on CRT response criteria is needed to compare outcomes of different studies and to be more conclusive.

Two small, single center studies also examined outcome of CRT in patients with a systemic right ventricle. Cecchin et al. included 9 patients (age 27 [0.5-43] years) and found a surprising high non-responding rate of 75% after a median follow-up duration of only 8 months (Cecchin et al. 2009). Cecchin et al. introduced additional criteria for identifying non-responders, namely patients with a decrease or <10% increase in systemic ejection fraction.

Jauvert et al. described outcomes of CRT therapy in 7 patients with CHD and a systemic right ventricle (age 24.6 [15-50] years) and observed clinical improvement in all patients. Mean NYHA class decreased from 3 to 1.6 and Vo2 max increased from 13.8 ± 2.5 to 22.8 ± 6.7 ml/kg/min. This study has the longest mean follow-up ($19.4m \pm 8.1$ months) of patients with a systemic right ventricle undergoing CRT (Janoušek et al. 2004).

Based on these relative small studies, CRT can be considered for patients in NYHA class $\geq$ II, impaired systemic right ventricular function and right bundle branch block, as recommended by the European working group on CHD (Budts et al. 2016). So far, studies have reported CRT outcome in a mixed population of adult and pediatric CHD patients. Association with clinical profiles, identification of risk factors for non-responders and the effect of systemic lead position could not be performed in these relative small studies. Hence, outcomes should be interpreted with caution. Key findings of all studies are summarized in Table 1.

Table 1. Studies on CRT in patients with SRV

Author	No. of SRV Pts	d-TGA (n,%)	cc-TGA (n,%)	No. of pts with available data	Age [range] (y)	M/F (n/n)	Fu [range] (y)	Clinical improvement (%)	Non-responders %	Mortality %	Comments
(Moore et al. 2019)	6	3 (50)	3 (50)	6	48 [36-73]	3/3	0.9 [0.2-1.9]	100	0	0	First report on hybrid transcatheter-surgical lead implantation in patients with SRV utilizing endocardial mapping to determine latest activation site.
(Flügge et al. 2018)	13	5 (38)	8 (62)	2	59.5 [50-69]	2/0	6.6 [3.2-10]	100	0	50	
(Koyak et al. 2018)	10	NA	NA	10	NA	NA	NA	60	40	NA	First study including only adults.
(Moore et al. 2018)	20	0	20 (100)	20	40 ± 15	10/10	4.6	67	33	0	First study focusing on technical considerations for lead implantation in cc-TGA.
(Karpawich et al. 2017)	8	6 (75)	2 (25)	8	28 [24-39]	8/0	2.7 [1-12]	100	NA	NA	Only patients with ≥15% increase of dP/dt-max after biventricular pacing underwent CRT implantation.
(Miyazaki et al. 2019, Miyazaki et al. 2015)	4	1 (25)	3 (75)	4	31.5 [9-47]	NA	4 [0.2-5.9]	0	100	0	In 2019 Miyazaki reports outcome of 8 SRV patients including patients from 2016. No data specified on this group, however they now report a non-responder rate of 50%.
(Yeo et al. 2014)	7	0	7 (100)	7	46 ± 10	NA	2 ± 1	NA	NA	NA	Data is not specified per patient, however significant improvement in mean NYHA class and SRV function was observed.

Table 1. (Continued)

Author	No. of SRV Pts	d-TGA (n,%)	cc-TGA (n,%)	No. of pts with available data	Age [range] (y)	M/F (n/n)	Fu [range] (y)	Clinical improvement (%)	Non-responders %	Mortality %	Comments
(Janoušek et al. 2009)	36	12 (33)	20 (56)	27	28.8	NA	0.6	NA	14	NA	Largest multicenter study. Data not specified per patient, however mean NYHA class and SRV function improved.
(Jauvert et al. 2009)	7	5 (71)	2 (29)	7	24.6 ± 12	4/3	1.6 ± 0.7	100	0	14	
(Cecchin et al. 2009)	9	NA	6 (67)	9	27 [0.5-43]	NA	>3 months	NA	67	22	First multicenter study on CRT in CHD.
(Dubin et al. 2005)	17	4 (24)	13 (76)	17	12.7 [4.9-50]	NA	NA	76	NA	0	
(Janoušek et al. 2004)	8	4 (50)	3 (38)	8	12.5 [7-29]	NA	1.5 [0.6-1.6]	NA	NA	0	First study reporting on outcomes of CRT in patients with SRV. Data not specified per patient, however mean NYHA class and SRV function improved.

cc-TGA = Congenitally corrected transposition of the great arteries, d-TGA = Dextro transposition of the great arteries, F = Female, Fu = Follow-up, M = Male, NA = Not available, NYHA = New York heart association, Pts = Patients, SRV = Systemic right ventricle, y = Year.

Table 2. Studies on multisite single ventricle pacing in Fontan patients

Author	No. of patients	Morphological RV (%)	No. of patients with available data	Age [range] (y)	Fu [range] (y)	Median number of leads [range]	Clinical improvement (%)	Non-responders (%)	Mortality (%)
(Cecchin et al. 2009)	13	NA	11	17.3 [0.5-42.5]	> 0.3 [0.3-1]	NA	91	9	15
(Janoušek et al. 2009)	4	25	4	10.3 [3.7-30.3]	1 [0-1.7]	2.5 [2-3]	75	25	0
(Dubin et al. 2005)	7	NA	7	3.1 [0.4-23.7]	NA	NA	29	57	NA

Fu = Follow-up, NA = Not available, Pts = Patients, RV = Right ventricle, y = Year.

Cardiac Resynchronization Therapy for the Failing Fontan

A Fontan circulation, constructed by staged repair, is the treatment of choice for children with single ventricle anatomy. The underlying anatomy and physiology are totally different compared to a biventricular circulation. Multiple reoperations, different types of Fontan-repair, elevated systemic venous blood pressure, non-pulsatile pulmonary blood flow and difference in systemic ventricular morphology create a unique population who is at high risk for development of heart failure. CRT can also be applied to patients with a Fontan circulation by multisite single ventricle pacing.

Several studies, which are summarized in Table 2, aimed at examining the acute hemodynamic effects of this pacing technique in the early post-operative setting. Initial results were promising, as hemodynamic parameters including blood pressure and cardiac index improved and QRS duration decreased after multisite single ventricle pacing.

No dedicated studies have reported on outcomes of CRT in patients with a Fontan circulation, although some studies focusing on CRT in CHD did include Fontan patients. The first study by Cecchin et al. included 13 single ventricle patients (age: 17.3 [0.5-42.5] years) and only 1 patient (9%) did not respond to CRT. Eight patients (62%) showed a 'strong' CRT response, which was defined as improvement in NYHA class by 2 or 3 points or an increase in EF ≥ 10 units. Two patients died during follow-up, one because of sudden cardiac death and one because of progressive heart failure. Another multicenter study included 4 Fontan patients (age 10.3 [3.7-30.3] years) and only 1 was a non-responder (Janoušek 2009). These promising results could not be substantiated by another multicenter study showing clinical improvement in only 2 out of 7 single ventricle patients (non-responders 71%) (Dubin et al. 2005).

Hence, current evidence for CRT in Fontan patients is scarce and inconsistent. There is no detailed information on e.g., the number and position of leads and differences in left and right ventricular morphology.

Future dedicated studies, ideally in a multicenter setting, are required to determine whether CRT is beneficial for patients with a Fontan circulation.

CURRENT SHORTCOMINGS AND FUTURE PERSPECTIVES

CRT can be an effective treatment modality for heart failure in adult patients with CHD. Current guidelines are cautious as evidence supporting CRT in this population has been limited to relatively small studies in which adults and pediatric patients with different underlying defects, including chanellopathies and cardiomyopathies, are included. Based on the results of these studies, the recent PACES/HRS Expert Consensus Statement on the Recognition and Management of Arrhyhtmias in Adult CHD has attempted to provide clinical guidance for this challenging population. However, these recommendations are mainly extrapolated from existing evidence for CRT in patients with ischemia induced heart failure.

Future studies are required to further elucidate and substantiate current guidelines. Uniform nomenclature on criteria to define 'responders' and 'non-responders' is essential to reliably compare study outcomes. By reporting outcomes of CRT in patients with CHD in a structured and homogenous manner, worldwide knowledge on its role in the treatment of heart failure will increase. Hence, we summarized the major limitations of current studies and provide future perspectives which will help us to accurately identify patient populations who are most likely to benefit from CRT:

- Multicenter studies should always be considered to include a sufficient number of adult/pediatric patients with similar underlying heart diseases.
- Distinction between pediatric and adult CHD patients is essential as CRT-response may be age related.
- Indications for CRT should be reported. Are we treating the failing systemic ventricle or are we aiming to 'prevent' (progression of) heart failure.

- Patients with systemic left ventricles, systemic right ventricles and patients with a Fontan circulation should be analyzed separately.
- Current studies mainly report on short-term outcomes of CRT in adult patients with CHD. Long-term outcomes of CRT need to be evaluated as well in order to determine the exact role of CRT in the treatment of heart failure in this specific population.
- Outcomes of CRT should include improvement in functional class (NYHA/Vo2 max etc.), hemodynamic echocardiographic changes (ventricular function, end-diastolic systemic ventricle diameter etc.) and alterations in QRS duration.
- Assessment of ventricular function can be challenging in this population due to abnormal ventricular geometry, previous cardiac surgery resulting in scar tissue and complex anatomical variations, such as a systemic right ventricle. If possible, a more accurate method, such as cardiac magnetic resonance imaging, should be considered to evaluate the effect on systemic ventricular function.
- Correlation of effectiveness of CRT and lead location is essential to determine optimal lead position. Furthermore, endocardial and/or epicardial mapping can localize the region of latest ventricular activation and areas of slow conduction, which are assumed to be the most optimal pacing sites to decrease interventricular dyssynchrony.
- Differences in effectiveness of CRT with either epicardial or transvenous leads is unknown.
- Sex differences in outcome of CRT in patients with CHD should be included (Hsich 2019).

REFERENCES

Abraham, W. T., W. G. Fisher, A. L. Smith, D. B. Delurgio, A. R. Leon, E. Loh, D. Z. Kocovic, M. Packer, A. L. Clavell, D. L. Hayes, M. Ellestad, R. J. Trupp, J. Underwood, F. Pickering, C. Truex, P. McAtee, J.

Messenger, and Miracle Study Group. Multicenter InSync Randomized Clinical Evaluation. 2002. "Cardiac resynchronization in chronic heart failure." *N Engl J Med* 346 (24):1845-53.

Budts, W., J. Roos-Hesselink, T. Radle-Hurst, A. Eicken, T. A. McDonagh, E. Lambrinou, M. G. Crespo-Leiro, F. Walker, and A. A. Frogoudaki. 2016. "Treatment of heart failure in adult congenital heart disease: a position paper of the Working Group of Grown-Up Congenital Heart Disease and the Heart Failure Association of the European Society of Cardiology." *Eur Heart J* 37 (18):1419-27.

Cecchin, F., P. A. Frangini, D. W. Brown, F. Fynn-Thompson, M. E. Alexander, J. K. Triedman, K. Gauvreau, E. P. Walsh, and C. I. Berul. 2009. "Cardiac resynchronization therapy (and multisite pacing) in pediatrics and congenital heart disease: Five years experience in a single institution." *J Cardiovasc Electrophysiol* 20 (1):58-65. doi:10.1 111/j.1 540-8167.2008.01274.x.

Dubin, A. M., J. Janousek, E. Rhee, M. J. Strieper, F. Cecchin, I. H. Law, K. M. Shannon, J. Temple, E. Rosenthal, F. J. Zimmerman, A. Davis, P. P. Karpawich, A. Al Ahmad, V. L. Vetter, N. J. Kertesz, M. Shah, C. Snyder, E. Stephenson, M. Emmel, S. Sanatani, R. Kanter, A. Batra, and K. K. Collins. 2005. "Resynchronization therapy in pediatric and congenital heart disease patients: An international multicenter study." *J Am Coll Cardiol* 46 (12):2277-2283. doi: 10.1016/j.jacc.2005.05.096.

Flügge, A. K., K. Wasmer, S. Orwat, H. Abdul-Khaliq, P. C. Helm, U. Bauer, H. Baumgartner, and G. P. Diller. 2018. "Cardiac resynchronization therapy in congenital heart disease: Results from the German National Register for Congenital Heart Defects." *Int J Cardiol* 273:108-111. doi: 10.1016/j.ijcard.2018.10.014.

Hsich, E. M. 2019. "Sex Differences in Advanced Heart Failure Therapies." *Circulation* 139 (8):1080-1093.

Janoušek, J. 2009. "Cardiac resynchronisation in congenital heart disease." *Heart* 95 (11):940-947. doi: 10.1136/hrt.2008.151266.

Janoušek, J., R. A. Gebauer, H. Abdul-Khaliq, M. Turner, L. Kornyei, O. Grollmuß, E. Rosenthal, E. Villain, A. Früh, T. Paul, N. A. Blom, J. M. Happonen, U. Bauersfeld, J. R. Jacobsen, F. Van Den Heuvel, T.

Delhaas, J. Papagiannis, and C. Trigo. 2009. "Cardiac resynchronisation therapy in paediatric and congenital heart disease: Differential effects in various anatomical and functional substrates." *Heart* 95 (14):1165-1171. doi: 10.1136/hrt.2008.160465.

Janousek, J., R. A. Gebauer, H. Abdul-Khaliq, M. Turner, L. Kornyei, O. Grollmuss, E. Rosenthal, E. Villain, A. Fruh, T. Paul, N. A. Blom, J. M. Happonen, U. Bauersfeld, J. R. Jacobsen, F. van den Heuvel, T. Delhaas, J. Papagiannis, C. Trigo, Dysrhythmias Working Group for Cardiac, and Cardiology Electrophysiology of the Association for European Paediatric. 2009. "Cardiac resynchronisation therapy in paediatric and congenital heart disease: differential effects in various anatomical and functional substrates." *Heart* 95 (14):1165-71.

Janoušek, J., V. Tomek, V. Chaloupecký, O. Reich, R. A. Gebauer, J. Kautzner, and B. Hučín. 2004. "Cardiac resynchronization therapy: A novel adjunct to the treatment and prevention of systemic right ventricular failure." *J Am Coll Cardiol* 44 (9):1927-1931. doi: 10.101 6/j.jacc.2004.08.044.

Jauvert, G., J. Rousseau-Paziaud, E. Villain, L. Iserin, F. Hidden-Lucet, M. Ladouceur, and D. Sidi. 2009. "Effects of cardiac resynchronization therapy on echocardiographic indices, functional capacity, and clinical outcomes of patients with a systemic right ventricle." *Europace* 11 (2):184-190. doi: 10.1093/europace/eun319.

Karpawich, P. P., N. Bansal, S. Samuel, Y. Sanil, and K. Zelin. 2017. "16 Years of Cardiac Resynchronization Pacing among Congenital Heart Disease Patients: Direct Contractility (dP/dt-max) Screening When the Guidelines Do Not Apply." *JACC Clin Electrophysiol* 3 (8):830-841.

Koyak, Z., J. R. De Groot, A. Krimly, T. M. MacKay, B. J. Bouma, C. K. Silversides, E. N. Oechslin, U. Hoke, L. Van Erven, W. Budts, I. C. Van Gelder, B. J. M. Mulder, and L. Harris. 2018. "Cardiac resynchronization therapy in adults with congenital heart disease." *Europace* 20 (2):315-322. doi: 10.1093/europace/euw386.

Marelli, A. J., R. Ionescu-Ittu, A. S. Mackie, L. Guo, N. Dendukuri, and M. Kaouache. 2014. "Lifetime prevalence of congenital heart disease in the general population from 2000 to 2010." *Circulation* 130 (9):749-56.

Miyazaki, A., J. Negishi, Y. Hayama, S. Baba, Y. Matsumura, Y. Shima, E. Tsuda, H. Sakaguchi, T. Hoashi, K. Kagisaki, T. Noda, H. Doi, H. Ichikawa, and H. Ohuchi. 2019. "Evaluating the response to cardiac resynchronization therapy performed with a new ventricular morphology-based strategy for congenital heart disease." *Heart Vessels* 34 (8):1340-1350. doi: 10.1007/s00380-019-01369-2.

Miyazaki, A., H. Sakaguchi, K. Kagisaki, N. Tsujii, M. Matsuoka, T. Yamamoto, T. Hoashi, T. Noda, and H. Ohuchi. 2015. "Optimal pacing sites for cardiac resynchronization therapy for patients with a systemic right ventricle with or without a rudimentary left ventricle." *Europace* 18 (1):100-112. doi: 10.1093/europace/euu401.

Moore, J. P., D. Cho, J. P. Lin, G. Lluri, L. C. Reardon, J. A. Aboulhosn, A. Hageman, and K. M. Shannon. 2018. "Implantation techniques and outcomes after cardiac resynchronization therapy for congenitally corrected transposition of the great arteries." *Heart Rhythm*. doi: 10.1016/j.hrthm.2018.08.017.

Moore, J. P., R. G. Gallotti, K. M. Shannon, and R. Biniwale. 2019. "A minimally invasive hybrid approach for cardiac resynchronization of the systemic right ventricle." *PACE Pacing Clin Electrophysiol* 42 (2):171-177. doi: 10.1111/pace.13568.

Moss, A. J., W. J. Hall, D. S. Cannom, H. Klein, M. W. Brown, J. P. Daubert, N. A. Estes, 3rd, E. Foster, H. Greenberg, S. L. Higgins, M. A. Pfeffer, S. D. Solomon, D. Wilber, W. Zareba, and Madit-Crt Trial Investigators. 2009. "Cardiac-resynchronization therapy for the prevention of heart-failure events." *N Engl J Med* 361 (14):1329-38.

Nieminen, H. P., E. V. Jokinen, and H. I. Sairanen. 2007. "Causes of late deaths after pediatric cardiac surgery: a population-based study." *J Am Coll Cardiol* 50 (13):1263-71.

Oechslin, E. N., D. A. Harrison, M. S. Connelly, G. D. Webb, and S. C. Siu. 2000. "Mode of death in adults with congenital heart disease." *Am J Cardiol* 86 (10):1111-6.

Ponikowski, P., A. A. Voors, S. D. Anker, H. Bueno, J. G. F. Cleland, A. J. S. Coats, V. Falk, J. R. Gonzalez-Juanatey, V. P. Harjola, E. A. Jankowska, M. Jessup, C. Linde, P. Nihoyannopoulos, J. T. Parissis, B.

Pieske, J. P. Riley, G. M. C. Rosano, L. M. Ruilope, F. Ruschitzka, F. H. Rutten, P. van der Meer, and E. S. C. Scientific Document Group. 2016. "2016 ESC Guidelines for the diagnosis and treatment of acute and chronic heart failure: The Task Force for the diagnosis and treatment of acute and chronic heart failure of the European Society of Cardiology (ESC)Developed with the special contribution of the Heart Failure Association (HFA) of the ESC." *Eur Heart J* 37 (27):2129-2200.

Tennant, P. W., M. S. Pearce, M. Bythell, and J. Rankin. 2010. "20-year survival of children born with congenital anomalies: a population-based study." *Lancet* 375 (9715):649-56.

van der Bom, T., A. C. Zomer, A. H. Zwinderman, F. J. Meijboom, B. J. Bouma, and B. J. Mulder. 2011. "The changing epidemiology of congenital heart disease." *Nat Rev Cardiol* 8 (1):50-60.

Yancy, C. W., M. Jessup, B. Bozkurt, J. Butler, D. E. Casey, Jr., M. M. Colvin, M. H. Drazner, G. S. Filippatos, G. C. Fonarow, M. M. Givertz, S. M. Hollenberg, J. Lindenfeld, F. A. Masoudi, P. E. McBride, P. N. Peterson, L. W. Stevenson, and C. Westlake. 2017. "2017 ACC/AHA/HFSA Focused Update of the 2013 ACCF/AHA Guideline for the Management of Heart Failure: A Report of the American College of Cardiology/American Heart Association Task Force on Clinical Practice Guidelines and the Heart Failure Society of America." *J Am Coll Cardiol* 70 (6):776-803.

Yeo, W. T., J. W. E. Jarman, W. Li, M. A. Gatzoulis, and T. Wong. 2014. "Adverse impact of chronic subpulmonary left ventricular pacing on systemic right ventricular function in patients with congenitally corrected transposition of the great arteries." *Int J Cardiol* 171 (2):184-191. doi: 10.1016/j.ijcard.2013.11.128.

Zomer, A. C., I. Vaartjes, E. T. van der Velde, H. M. de Jong, T. C. Konings, L. J. Wagenaar, W. F. Heesen, F. Eerens, L. H. Baur, D. E. Grobbee, and B. J. Mulder. 2013. "Heart failure admissions in adults with congenital heart disease; risk factors and prognosis." *Int J Cardiol* 168 (3):2487-93.

BIOGRAPHICAL SKETCHES

Rohit K. Kharbanda

Affiliation: Erasmus Medical Center, Rotterdam, the Netherlands

Education: Medical doctor, research fellow cardiothoracic surgery – Cardiology Electrophysiology

Business Address: Doctor Molewaterplein 40

Research and Professional Experience: Research fellow

Professional Appointments: NA

Honors: Master degree in medicine with honor

Publications from the Last 3 Years:

1. Kharbanda RK, Özdemir EH, Taverne YJHJ, et al. Current concepts of anatomy, electrophysiology, and therapeutic implications of the interatrial septum. *JACC Clin Electrophysiol* 5(6): 647-656.
2. Kharbanda RK, de Groot NMS. Prediction and prevention of sudden cardiac death in transposition of the great arteries: A step closer. *Int J Cardiol* 2019;1;288:68-69.
3. Kharbanda RK, Garcia-Izquierdo E, Bogers A, De Groot NMS. Focal activation patterns: breaking new grounds in the pathophysiology of atrial fibrillation. *Expert Rev Cardiovasc Ther* 2018;16:479-88.
4. Kharbanda RK, Blom NA, Hazekamp MG, et al. Incidence and risk factors of post-operative arrhythmias and sudden cardiac death after atrioventricular septal defect (AVSD) correction: Up to 47years of follow-up. *Int J Cardiol* 2018;252:88-93.

5. van Rosendael AR, de Graaf MA, Dimitriu-Leen AC, et al. The influence of clinical and acquisition parameters on the interpretability of adenosine stress myocardial computed tomography perfusion. *Eur Heart J Cardiovasc Imaging* 2017;18:203-11.

Ad J.J.C. Bogers

Affiliation: Erasmus Medical Center, Rotterdam, the Netherlands

Education: Medical doctor, cardiothoracic surgeon

Business Address: Doctor Molewaterplein 40

Research and Professional Experience: Professor in cardiothoracic surgery, specialized in pediatric and adult congenital heart surgery

Professional Appointments: Cardiothoracic surgeon, Erasmus Medical Center, head of cardiothoracic surgery department

Honors: XXX

Publications from the Last 3 Years:

1. Teuwen CP, Yaksh A, Lanter EA, Kik C, van der Does LJ, Knops P, Taverne YJ, van de Woestijne PC, Oei FB, Bekkers JA, Bogers AJ, Allessie MA, De Groot NM. Relevance of Conduction Disorders in Bachmann's Bundle During Sinus Rhythm in Humans. *Circ Arrhythm Electrophysiol*. 2016.
2. de Groot, NMS, van der Does LJ, Yaksh A, Lanters EA, Teuwen CP, Knops P, van de Woestijne PC, Bekkers JA, Kik C, Bogers AJ, Allessie MA. Direct Proof of Endo-Epicardial Asynchrony of the

Atrial Wall During Atrial Fibrillation in Humans. *Circ Arrhythm Electrophysiol.*, 2016.
3. Mouws EMJP, Lanters EAH, Teuwen CP, van der Does LJME, Kik C, Knops P, Bekkers JA, Bogers AJJC, de Groot NMS. Epicardial Breakthrough Waves During Sinus Rhythm: Depiction of the Arrhythmogenic Substrate? *Circ Arrhythm Electrophysiol.* 2017.
4. Kharbanda RK, Özdemir EH, Taverne YJHJ, et al. Current concepts of anatomy, electrophysiology, and therapeutic implications of the interatrial septum. *JACC Clin Electrophysiol* 5(6): 647-656.

Natasja MS de Groot

Affiliation: Erasmus Medical Center, Rotterdam, the Netherlands

Education: Medical doctor, cardiologist-electrophysiologist

Business Address: Doctor Molewaterplein 40

Research and Professional Experience: Professor in Electrophysiology

Professional Appointments: cardiologist-electrophysiologist Erasmus Medical Center, chief unit translational electrophysiology.

Honors: Female Hero in Science, VIDI (Dutch Academy of Sciences), Fellow of the European Heart Rhythm Association

Publications from the Last 3 Years:

1. Teuwen CP, Yaksh A, Lanter EA, Kik C, van der Does LJ, Knops P, Taverne YJ, van de Woestijne PC, Oei FB, Bekkers JA, Bogers AJ, Allessie MA, De Groot NM. Relevance of Conduction

Disorders in Bachmann's Bundle during Sinus Rhythm in Humans. *Circ Arrhythm Electrophysiol.* 2016.
2. de Groot, NMS, van der Does LJ, Yaksh A, Lanters EA, Teuwen CP, Knops P, van de Woestijne PC, Bekkers JA, Kik C, Bogers AJ, Allessie MA. Direct Proof of Endo-Epicardial Asynchrony of the Atrial Wall During Atrial Fibrillation in Humans. *Circ Arrhythm Electrophysiol.*, 2016.
3. Mouws EMJP, Lanters EAH, Teuwen CP, van der Does LJME, Kik C, Knops P, Bekkers JA, Bogers AJJC, de Groot NMS. Epicardial Breakthrough Waves during Sinus Rhythm: Depiction of the Arrhythmogenic Substrate? *Circ Arrhythm Electrophysiol.* 2017.
4. Unipolar atrial electrogram morphology from an epicardial and endocardial perspective. van der Does LJME, Knops P, Teuwen CP, Serban C, Starreveld R, Lanters EAH, Mouws EMJP, Kik C, Bogers AJJC, de Groot NMS. *Heart Rhythm.* 2018 Jun;15(6):879-887
5. Zhang D, Hu X, Li J, Liu J, Baks-Te Bulte L, Wiersma M, Malik NU, van Marion DMS, Tolouee M, Hoogstra-Berends F, Lanters EAH, van Roon AM, de Vries AAF, Pijnappels DA, de Groot NMS, Henning RH, Brundel BJJM. DNA damage-induced PARP1 activation confers cardiomyocyte dysfunction through NAD_+ depletion in experimental atrial fibrillation. *Nat Commun.* 2019 Mar 21;10(1):1307.

In: Congenital Heart Disease
Editor: Curtis Giguère
ISBN: 978-1-53616-674-3
© 2020 Nova Science Publishers, Inc.

Chapter 4

TYPES, PRESENTATION, AND MANAGEMENT OF ATRIAL SEPTAL DEFECTS IN ADULTS

Samantha Whitwell, Frank Han, MD,
Michael McMullan, MD and William Campbell, MD*
University of Mississippi Medical Center, Jackson, MS, US

INCIDENCE AND ETIOLOGY

There are four different types of atrial septal defects (ASDs) categorized based on location and embryological development. While the bicuspid aortic valve is the most common congenital heart anomaly in adults, ASDs are not far behind, accounting for 10-15% of congenital heart disease [5, 6]. They also account for approximately 100 of 100 000 live births in the current era of echocardiography. While some familial conditions, such as Holt-Oram syndrome are associated with ASDs, the inheritance pattern is mostly unknown. Other syndromes associated with atrial septal defects include Down Syndrome, Ellis van Creveld Syndrome, and Digeorge Syndrome.

---

[*] Corresponding Author's Email: fhan01@gmail.com.

Within the spectrum of atrial septal defects, the secundum subtype is the most common (~75%), followed by the ostium primum, sinus venosus, and coronary sinus atrial septal defects.

EMBRYOLOGY

The atria begin as a large common chamber in the early fetus [1]. At approximately the fourth week of gestation, the septum primum comes down from the roof of the common atrium and builds a barrier that eventually connects to the endocardial cushion, the structure that will form the AV node and division between the mitral and tricuspid valve. The hole that is formed during this process is the ostium primum. Before the septum is completely formed, the upper part of the septum primum begins to experience apoptosis, which creates the "second hole," or the ostium secundum. It is important to note that the ostium secundum atrial septal defect, which will be introduced shortly, is not a defect in the septum secundum, despite the similar naming scheme. The formation of the septum primum occurs between the fifth and six weeks of fetal life. The next division occurs when the septum secundum appears, to the anatomic right side of the first septum. This septum grows inwards from the superior and inferior aspects of the right atrium. It does not entirely seal over, instead, it leaves a small communication on its inferior aspect. The communication between the right atrium, septum secundum, and septum primum, is termed the oval foramen, which allows normal fetal right to left shunting prior to birth.

MORPHOLOGY AND CLASSIFICATION

Atrial septal defects come in many shapes and sizes, and can also be multi-fenestrated. The four primary categories of atrial septal defects are the sinus venosus defect, the ostium primum atrial septal defect, ostium secundum atrial septal defect, and the unroofed coronary sinus. The names are derived from the defect in the embryologic formation of the atrial septum, as noted in Figure 1. All defects produce a left to right shunt depending on the size of the hole, the presence of elevated pulmonary vascular resistance, and the compliance of the atria, but the clinical features and unique features in their diagnosis are important. Generally, these defects initially result in left to right shunting after birth. However, right to left shunting can occur in the setting of elevated right heart pressures. The presence of additional heart lesions such as pulmonary valve stenosis and pulmonary hypertension will further affect the net direction of blood flow across the ASD. The difference between these atrial septal defects will be described next.

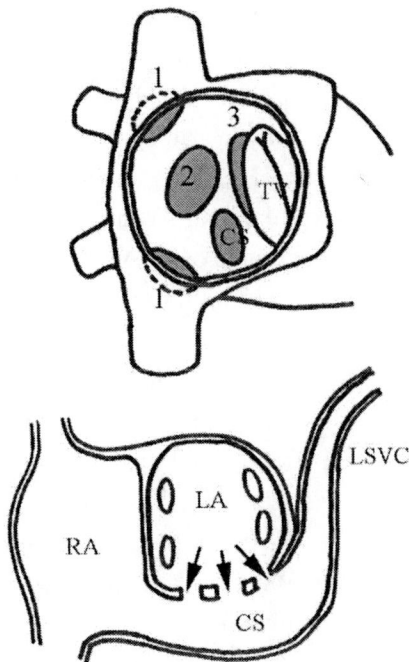

Figure 1. A schematic representation of the types of ASD. 1 = sinus venosus ASD. 2 = ostium secundum ASD. 3 = ostium primum ASD. TV = tricuspid valve. CS = coronary sinus. RA = right atrium. LA = left atrium. CS = coronary sinus. LSVC = left superior caval vein. The arrows illustrate defects in the roof of the coronary sinus which are the "unroofed" coronary sinus or coronary sinus atrial septal defect.

The sinus venosus defect is a septal defect that is located near the superior or inferior caval vein. All these defects represent the ostia of at least one pulmonary vein. The embryologic sinus venosus is a large sinus that represents the confluence of all venous tributaries. The right side of this structure merges into the wall of the right atrium, and the left side of this structure, through asymmetric expression of sidedness proteins, is the progenitor of the coronary sinus. Anomalous connection of a pulmonary vein onto the atrial septum generates the so-called sinus venosus atrial septal defect. Therefore, the defect is not a true hole in the atrial septum, but an orifice of a pulmonary vein.

The ostium primum atrial septal defect is located adjacent to the tricuspid and mitral valves, in an anatomically inferior location. These are part of the spectrum of atrioventricular septal defects (AVSD). The embryologic cause of this defect is the failure of the fusion of the "first wall" or septum primum, with the endocardial cushion. The alignment of the tricuspid and mitral valves in the same plane is a diagnostic clue of a potential ostium primum atrial septal defect, if not the presence of a complete atrioventricular septal defect – if further imaging demonstrates the other associated findings diagnostic of an AVSD.

The ostium secundum atrial septal defect is the most common form of atrial septal defect. It represents approximately 75% of all atrial septal defects. The embryologic cause of this defect is excessive resorption of the septum primum (primary septum). Such defects vary in size and can be fenestrated, or have multiple openings. This defect is located nearer to the center of the definitive atrial septum. The naming of the septal defect is a reference to its location near the embryologic secondary septal defect, rather than the secondary septum. When this is found in association with mitral stenosis (which itself is usually rheumatic in origin), the lesion is termed Lutembacher syndrome.

The unroofed coronary sinus is a defect in the roof of the coronary sinus which allows venous blood to mix with arterial blood at the level of the left atrium. There are four classifications of the unroofed coronary sinus: Type 1 is the completely unroofed coronary sinus with a persistent connection to a left superior caval vein (LSVC), Type 2 is the completely unroofed coronary sinus without a persistent LSVC, Type 3 is a coronary sinus that is partially unroofed in the mid-portion, and type 4 is a coronary sinus that is partially unroofed in the terminal portion. The left superior caval vein should be distinguished from the persistent left anterior cardinal vein, by tracing the venous blood flow. A left superior caval vein always passes anterior to the left pulmonary artery, whereas the persistent left sided anterior cardinal vein always passes posterior to the left pulmonary artery.

CLINICAL FINDINGS

The overall clinical findings depend on the net shunted blood flow. This in turn depends on the number of defects, their size, the compliance of the atria, and the presence of elevated pulmonary vascular resistance. The presentation will also vary by age. In infancy, even large atrial septal defects may cause only mild symptoms such as tachypnea with feeds, or even nothing at all. Toddlers and young children may be referred solely for the presence of a murmur upon physical examination. Typically, varying degrees of heart failure symptoms only occur when the patient is a teenager or a young adult. Older adults sometimes present with pulmonary hypertension, which must be evaluated prior to consideration for atrial septal defect closure. It is rare however, to find patients with atrial septal defects and Eisenmenger syndrome.

Small atrial septal defects may produce no physical examination findings. When the atrial septal defect starts producing a significant shunt, or when the ratio of pulmonary blood flow starts to exceed systemic blood flow by greater than 150%, a murmur due to increased flow across the pulmonary valve can be heard. In most cases the pulmonary valve will itself be normal, but the introduction of greatly increased flow across even a normal valve will generate a murmur. In atrial septal defects with significant shunting, the healthcare provider will be able to auscultate a fixed split S2. Determination of whether the patient has a fixed split S2, a widely split S2, or a respiratory split S2, will require careful comparison of the second heart sounds in inspiration and expiration.

Figure 2. The behavior of the second heart sound in inspiration versus expiration during normal respiratory splitting. The time between A2 and P2 extends with inspiration.

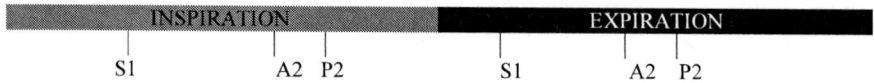

Figure 3. The behavior of the second heart sound in inspiration versus expiration during fixed respiratory splitting. No significant difference in time elapsed exists between the aortic and pulmonary sounds.

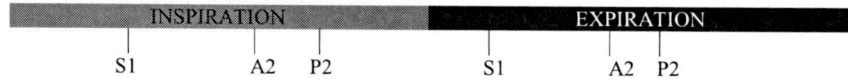

Figure 4. The behavior of the second heart sound in inspiration versus expiration during wide splitting. A baseline delay exists between the aortic and pulmonary sounds, and further extends during inspiration.

Atrial septal defects will produce an abnormal S2 by two primary mechanisms (Figures 2-4). The volume overload generated on the right ventricle will produce right atrial and right ventricular stretch. The stretch will then dilate the right ventricle, which will stretch the total length of the right bundle. When the right bundle experiences enough stretch, it will require more time to depolarize than the left anterior and posterior bundles. When this happens, varying degrees of right bundle branch block occur, and allow the right and left ventricles to experience a delay in their respective depolarizations. It is important to note that there is usually no intrinsic bundle branch disease in a patient with an uncomplicated ASD. The bundle branch block is rather a reflection of the increased distance traveled by the depolarizing current. The other mechanism of the fixed split S2 is the effect of the increased blood flow on the timing of the closure of the pulmonary valve. When we take a deep breath, bronchiolar and alveolar expansion to accommodate inspired air will exert pressure on the adjacent blood vessels. The pressure on the blood vessels will then generate transiently increased venous return to the right ventricle, which will then hold the pulmonary valve open longer than in the expiratory state. Thus, the P2 component will be delayed and the second heart sound will split. When a significant atrial septal defect is present, there is constant volume overload of the right ventricle. The constant volume overload of the right ventricle causes a constant degree of delay of the pulmonary component of the second heart sound, thus producing the auscultatory findings in Figure 3. The right bundle branch block can also contribute if the QRS duration is significantly lengthened.

DIAGNOSIS, INVESTIGATIONS, AND STUDIES

Electrocardiograms done on patients with small atrial septal defects are most often normal. Electrocardiograms done on patients with large atrial septal defects may produce varying degrees of right ventricular hypertrophy, right axis deviation, and right bundle branch block. An important exception to these guidelines is the primum atrial septal defect. As these defects exist along a spectrum of congenital heart disease known as the atrioventricular septal defects, the atrioventricular node is commonly located in an abnormal position. Thus, these septal defects are known to produce left axis or severe left axis deviation related to the abnormal average vector of ventricular depolarization.

The standard test for the diagnosis of atrial septal defects is the transthoracic echocardiogram. It is essential to define the entire atrial septum as certain patients may have more than one type of defect. In infants and small children, this test produces adequate windows to diagnose all types of atrial septal defect and their boundaries. Transesophageal echocardiography is only used in infants and young children as a perioperative tool for confirmation of complete closure of the defect and proper de-airing of the heart before termination of bypass. It is not usually used for the initial diagnosis due to the anesthesia risks. Transesophageal echocardiogram in small infants in certain scenarios may even produce worse spatial resolution than the transthoracic echocardiogram. Transesophageal echocardiogram could be necessary in the diagnosis of an atrial septal defect in the adult if the sonographic windows are limited.

Fetal echocardiography can assist in diagnosing atrial septal defects, but the diagnosis of small atrial septal defects is harder to make during fetal life because of the expected presence of a patent foramen ovale [2, 4]. Multiple views are typically required to ascertain that the fetus possesses an abnormal atrial septal communication.

In adults, especially with sinus venosus atrial septal defects, the size and boundaries of the defect are typically not easy to visualize secondary to body habitus and limited acoustic windows. Adult cardiologists often need to make use of agitated saline echocardiographic contrast or the transesophageal echocardiogram, to achieve the spatial resolution needed to diagnose these defects. One of the common reasons for referral is right heart dilation of unknown etiology. The presence of an ASD should be in the differential diagnosis of all patients with right heart dilation of undetermined etiology. The other pitfall to avoid is the false positive diagnosis of atrial septal defects on apical four chamber imaging in adult echocardiography. The lack of a clear view of the atrial septum in apical four chamber imaging can sometimes be mistaken for a septal defect. Other views must be obtained to confirm the presence of an atrial septal defect. The subcostal views are most helpful for this. If a sinus venosus atrial septal defect is found, a search must be initiated for each pulmonary vein, as the sinus venosus defect is not a true "atrial septal defect," rather it is the orifice of an abnormally connecting pulmonary vein. Identification of a sinus venosus atrial septal defect along with an abnormal pulmonary venous connection is termed partial anomalous pulmonary venous return (PAPVR).

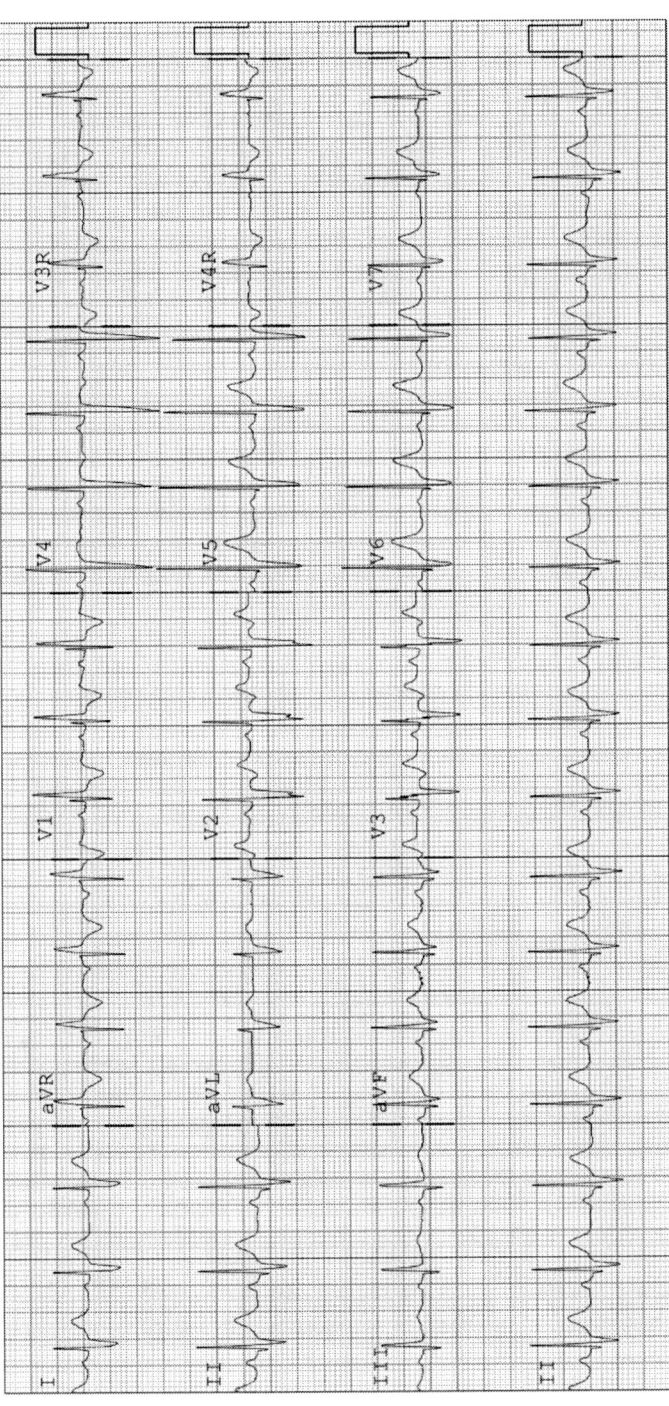

Figure 5. The EKG of a 5-year-old asymptomatic boy referred for a murmur, later found to have a large secundum atrial septal defect. The EKG demonstrates sinus rhythm, right axis deviation, and an incomplete right bundle branch block.

84 Samantha Whitwell, Frank Han, Michael McMullan et al.

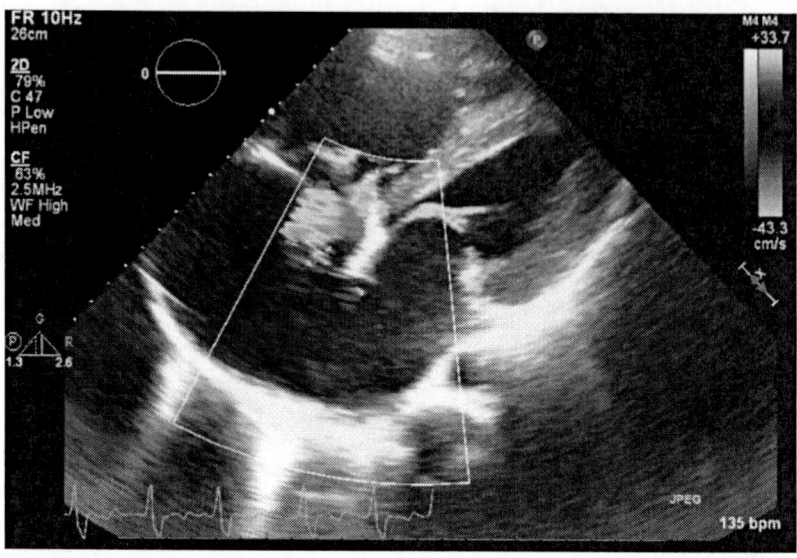

Figure 6. Transthoracic echocardiographic image of a secundum atrial septal defect. There is also four chamber dilation, mitral regurgitation, and tricuspid valve regurgitation. This 37-year-old adult male was in atrial fibrillation at the time of the study.

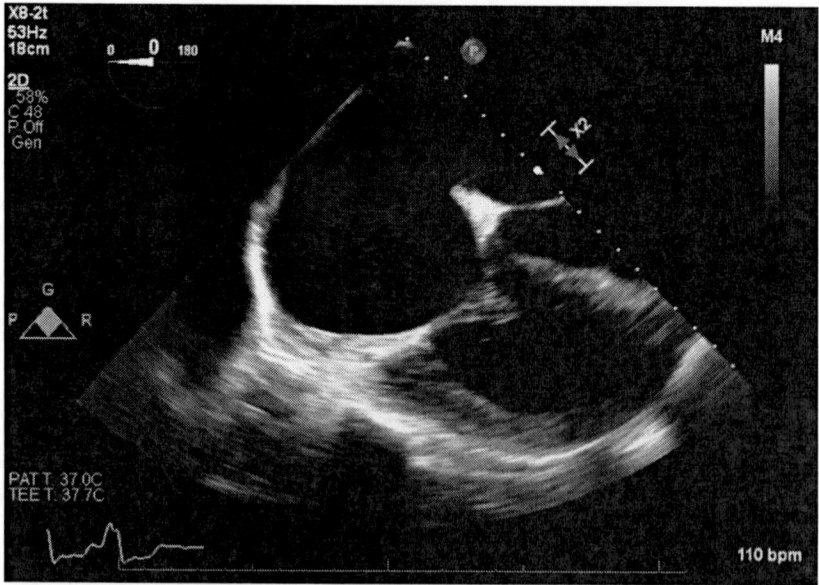

Figure 7. A transesophageal echocardiographic image of the same 37-year-old patient clearly confirming the presence of the large secundum atrial septal defect.

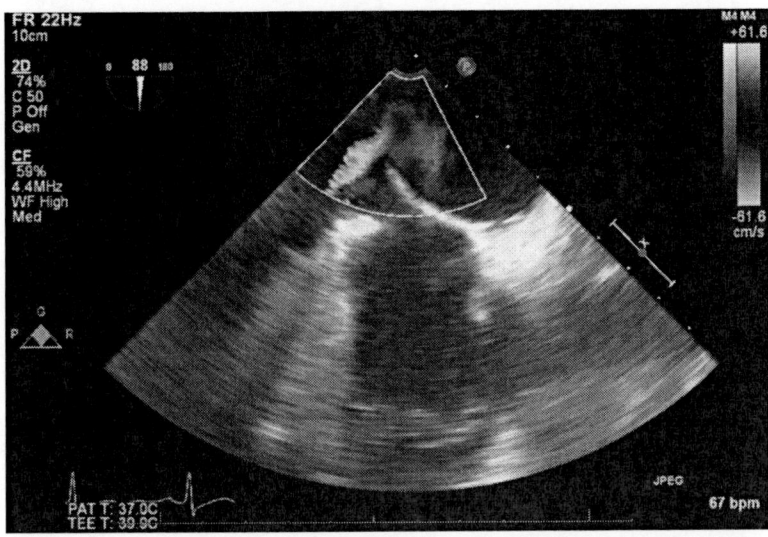

Figure 8. A transesophageal echocardiographic image of a 45-year-old male with an inferior sinus venosus atrial septal defect. This patient was referred for cardiac evaluation because of persistent cardiac symptoms despite previous secundum atrial septal defect closure. His pulmonary veins all returned normally.

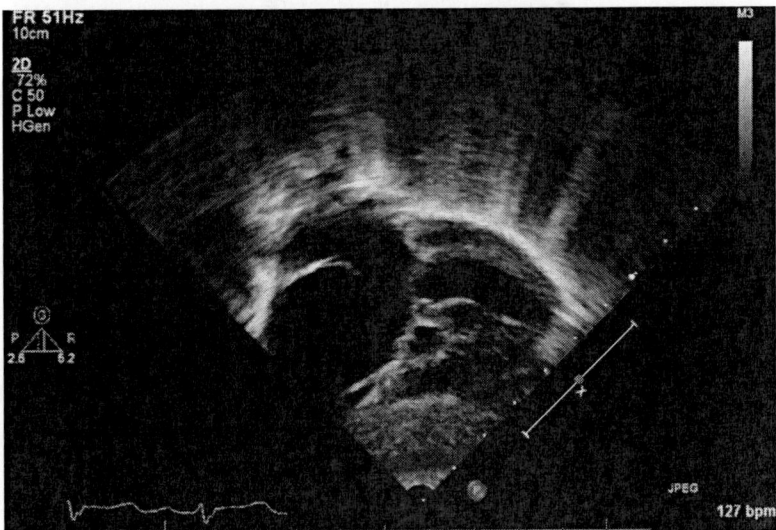

Figure 9. A transthoracic echocardiographic image of a 4-month-old infant with Down Syndrome and complete AV canal. The image illustrates the ostium primum atrial septal defect component of the complete atrioventricular canal. The presence of both AV valves on exactly the same plane also confirms the diagnosis of a complete AV canal.

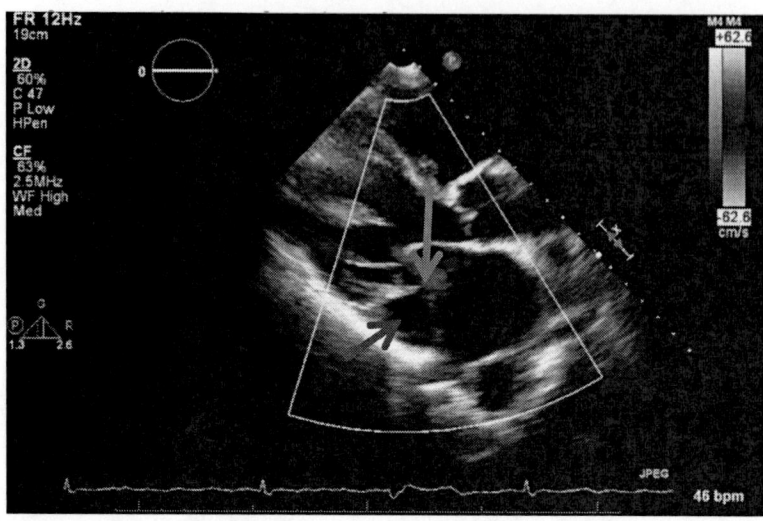

Figure 10. The unroofed coronary sinus atrial septal defect. Transthoracic echocardiographic imaging in parasternal long axis orientation in this 52-year-old male who was referred for new onset congestive heart failure and atrial fibrillation after prior atrial septal defect surgery as a younger man. The red arrow (more inferior) illustrates the markedly dilated coronary sinus which connects to a left sided superior vena cava (not shown in this image). The blue arrow (more superior) illustrates the unroofed portion of the coronary sinus. Mild aortic insufficiency is also present.

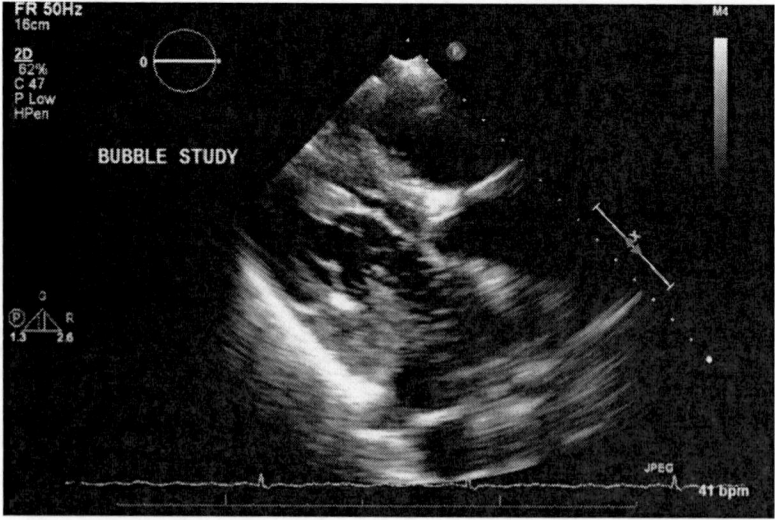

Figure 11. Agitated saline contrast study in the same patient done from the left arm, illustrating rapid entry of contrast into the left atrium prior to opacification of the right atrium.

TREATMENT

As an adult, a patient with an unrepaired atrial septal defect may present initially with atrial fibrillation with varying degrees of ventricular response. The initial presentation may also involve varying degrees of heart failure symptoms. Medical management in these patients depends on associated complications. Arrhythmias should be treated with anticoagulation, rate control, and possible synchronized cardioversion. ASD closure is recommended in patients with impaired function, including left-to-right shunting and right heart enlargement with or without symptoms, and in patients with paradoxical embolus or infectious endocarditis. A shunt run demonstrating pulmonary blood flow exceeding systemic blood flow by 150% or more is an indication for surgery [3]. This may also be expressed as a Q_p/Q_s ratio greater than or equal to 1.5:1.

The size of the ASD and the degree of the shunt directs the surgical management of patients with atrial septal defects. Very small defects often spontaneously close before the age of 5. If these defects persist into adulthood, left-to-right shunting will often worsen, leading to further complications and often require surgical repair. Surgical ablations of arrhythmias can be performed at the same time as atrial septal defect closure if necessary. Repair of the ostium primum atrial septal defect involves patch closure of the defect. As these are AVSDs, careful examination of the mitral valve is required to see if there is a cleft. If that is present, the cleft must also be closed. This type of defect is also repaired in conjunction with the complete AV canal. Repair of the ostium secundum atrial septal defect involves patch closure of the hole. Secundum ASDs can be closed in the catheterization laboratory if they have adequate surrounding rims. Device closure of certain sinus venosus atrial septal defects is also a newer repair technique; however this has not been fully adopted as standard of care yet [7]. Repair of the sinus venosus atrial septal defect usually involves baffled patch closure of the atrial septal defect to simultaneously redirect the anomalously connecting pulmonary vein and close the septal defect. Repair of the unroofed coronary sinus septal defect also involves patch closure of the defect.

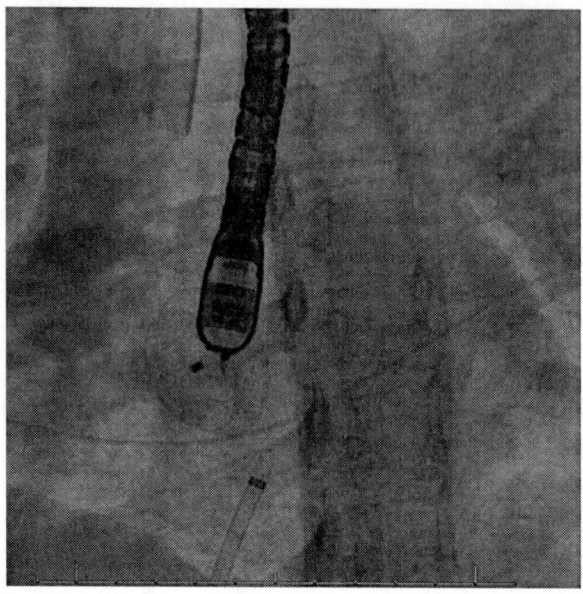

Figure 12. An image taken in the catheterization laboratory illustrating device closure of an atrial septal defect in a 23-year-old female who initially presented for cardiac evaluation due to chest pain and dyspnea on exertion. The device has been detached from its delivery system and is in good position.

ASD closure is contraindicated as a single procedure in patients that have developed pulmonary hypertension or Eisenmenger syndrome due to the risk of acute right heart failure. Such patients require diagnosis and treatment for pulmonary artery hypertension prior to consideration of closure of the atrial septal defect.

LONG TERM FOLLOWUP

Long term followup of the patient with a repaired atrial septal defect depends on the initial presenting conditions. If the patient was a teenager, young adult, or child who received a secundum atrial septal defect closure, and there are no residual lesions, the followup is rather infrequent. Occasionally, patch leaks may be encountered, but small ones do not require a repeat operation. Such patients rarely require any secondary intervention.

Patients who received closure of an ostium primum atrial septal defect with closure of a mitral valve cleft periodically develop left atrioventricular (mitral) valve stenosis or insufficiency, which sometimes requires a repeat operation. If the patient was an adult who presented with pulmonary hypertension, a treatment course of pulmonary hypertension would have been indicated prior to surgical repair. The surgical repair does not necessarily create immediate resolution of the pulmonary hypertension. The same applies to preoperative arrhythmias, which may not completely resolve after surgery. Therefore, long term followup with careful medication titration is necessary in that group of patients. If the patient received a sinus venosus atrial septal defect repair, a search for postoperative pulmonary vein stenosis, superior caval vein stenosis, and patch leaks must be completed. The combination of lesions depends on whether the patient required an SVC translocation (Warden Procedure) due to a remote insertion of the native pulmonary vein, or a simple patch baffle of the anomalously connecting pulmonary vein. There also is the occasional adult who was diagnosed with one type of atrial septal defect, who fails to achieve symptomatic relief after surgical repair. Such a patient presentation should raise the index of suspicion for a second undiagnosed atrial septal defect or associated lesions.

REFERENCES

[1] Fyler D. C.: Nadas' Pediatric Cardiology. Philadelphia: Hanley and Belfus, 1992.

[2] Hubail Z., Lemler M., Ramaciotti C., Moore J., Ikemba C. Diagnosing a Patent Foramen Ovale in Children – Is Transesophageal Echocardiography necessary? *Stroke* 2011; 42:98-101.

[3] Horvath K. A., Burke R. P., Collins J. J., and Cohn L. H.: Surgical treatment of adult atrial septal defect: Early and long-term results. *J. Am. Coll. Cardiol.* 1992; 20: pp. 1156-1159.

[4] Razdan S., Strouse J., Naik R., Lanzkron S., Urrutia V., Resar J. et al. Patent Foramen Ovale in Patients with Sickle Cell Disease and Stroke: Case Presentations and Review of the Literature.

[5] Sutton, Martin G. "Clinical manifestations and diagnosis of atrial septal defects in adults." *UpToDate,* 2018. Accessed April 2019.
[6] Botto L. D., Correa A., Erickson J. D. Racial and temporal variations in the prevalence of heart defects. *Pediatrics* 2001;107: E32.
[7] Thakkar, A. N., Chinnadurai, P., Breinholt, J. P., & Lin, C. H. (2018). Transcatheter closure of a sinus venosus atrial septal defect using 3D printing and image fusion guidance. *Catheterization and Cardiovascular Interventions, 92*(2), 353-357. doi:10.1002/ccd.27645

In: Congenital Heart Disease
Editor: Curtis Giguère

ISBN: 978-1-53616-674-3
© 2020 Nova Science Publishers, Inc.

Chapter 5

STATE OF THE LIVER IN CHILDREN WITH CONGENITAL HEART DISEASE

M. P. Lymarenko
Department of Pediatrics,
Faculty of Internship and Postgraduate Education,
Donetsk National Medical University named after M. Gorky, Ukraine

ABSTRACT

Congenital heart disease (CHD) – one of the most common congenital anomalies in children (30% of all congenital malformations); in terms of frequency of occurrence, it ranks third after congenital pathology of the musculoskeletal system and central nervous system.

It should be noted that in diseases of the heart, including congenital heart disease, the liver is affected due to an acute or chronic increase in central venous pressure, as well as a decrease in cardiac output. The phenomena of stagnation, necrosis, fibrosis, less often cirrhosis, which may exist separately, but are often combined depending on the clinical situation, are usually observed. To refer to these disorders, a number of authors suggest the term «cardiogenic liver».

In the medical literature there are very few reports on the state of the liver, cholestatic disorders in children with congenital heart disease. Most publications concern Alagille syndrome.

The purpose of our research was to study the state of the liver in children with congenital heart disease and chronic heart failure. We observed 45 children. Congenital heart disease represented: ventricular septal defect – in 26,7% of patients, secondary atrial septal defect – in 24,4% of children, a double discharge of the main vessels of the right ventricle – in 15,6% of patients, common atrioventricular canal – at 15,6% of children, tetralogy of Fallot – at 11,1% of patients, etc. Combined congenital heart disease were diagnosed in 17,8% of children. Hepatosplenomegaly without liver dysfunction was found in 75,6% of patients. In all cases, enlargement of the liver associated with hemodynamic compromise and venous stagnation of blood in it.

Keywords: congenital heart disease, liver, children

Cardiovascular diseases constitute one of the leading sections of the pathology of childhood and lead to a high disability of the child population and mortality. In recent decades, along with a decrease in the incidence of rheumatism and, consequently, the frequency of the formation of acquired heart defects, the congenital pathology of the heart and great vessels, which is initially the cause of early disability and child mortality, especially in the first year of life, has become increasingly relevant.

Congenital heart disease (CHD) – one of the most common congenital anomalies in children (30% of all congenital malformations); in terms of frequency of occurrence, it ranks third after congenital pathology of the musculoskeletal system and central nervous system [1-3]. CHD are found, according to various authors [2, 3], in 0,7 - 1,7% of newborns. In recent years there has been an increase in this indicator, probably due to the use of more advanced methods of functional diagnostics and an increased interest in the problem of CHD of other specialties. Thus, up to 30–35 thousand children with CHD are born each year in the USA, and 20–22 thousand children in Russia [1-3].

In the structure of congenital heart disease [3], about half of them are due to defects with enrichment of the pulmonary circulation (ventricular septal defect (VSD), atrial septal defect (ASD), patent ductus arteriosus (PDA), total anomalous pulmonary venous connection, common atrioventricular canal, etc.). Most of them are acinotic CHD. The smaller group consists of cyanotic CHD with venous-arterial blood discharge and depletion of the pulmonary circulation (tetralogy of Fallot, Ebstein's anomaly, transposition of the great arteries, pulmonic stenosis with VSD, etc.).

Approximately in ⅓ of cases, CHD is combined with extracardiac congenital anomalies of the musculoskeletal system, central nervous system, gastrointestinal tract, urinary system [3, 4]. If large extracardiac malformations affecting the course of CHD are diagnosed in almost 70% of patients, then minor developmental anomalies, or stigmas, are found in more than 40% of patients. At the same time, the presence of more than 3-5 stigmas of diembriogenesis increases the probability of detecting CHD [2].

In the etiology of CHD, three major factors are unconditional [3]: genetic inheritance of the defect; the impact of environmental factors that have a pathological effect on embryogenesis with the formation of embryo- and fetopathy; a combination of genetic predisposition and pathological effects of various environmental factors. Genetic inheritance of the defect can be caused by both quantitative and structural chromosomal aberrations (5%), as well as mutation of a single gene (2-3%). Among the environmental factors, first of all, intraoral viral infections should be distinguished, i.e., viral infections transmitted in the first trimester of pregnancy. The teratogenic role of rubella, coxsackie, chicken pox, herpes simplex viruses, adenoviruses, cytomegalovirus viruses, causative agents of toxoplasmosis, mycoplasmosis, listeriosis, syphilis, tuberculosis has been proven [2, 3]. Other risk factors for having a child with CHD include: endocrine diseases, especially diabetes in the mother; maternal alcoholism; taking a number of drugs (hydantoin, trimetadion, difenin, amphetamines, lithium preparations, etc.) by women in the early stages of pregnancy; occupational hazards-work with paints, varnishes, gasoline; severe toxicosis of the first half of pregnancy, etc.

Introduction to clinical practice of a large number of modern, constantly updated methods of research of the cardiovascular system (three-dimensional sectoral echocardiography with color mapping, color doppler echocardiography, nuclear magnetic resonance, Holter monitoring, electrophysiological examination of the heart, catheterization and angiocardiography) and improvement of routine methods, orthogonal electrocardiogram (ECG), multipolar ECG, large-scale ECG, transesophageal ECG, and immunological and genetic research methods significantly increased the diagnostic capabilities of the doctor [3].

It should be emphasized that the tremendous progress achieved in the surgery of congenital heart disease, the development of endovascular surgery not only saved the sick children with seemingly incompatible defects, but also prolonged their life for many years. The contingent of patients with complex multicomponent CHD is constantly increasing, which means that the pediatric cardiologist must be able to correctly diagnose them, perform an extensive set of measures for the preoperative management of such patients, know the indications for prescribing surgical treatment, the timing and nature of palliative and radical reconstructive operations. He also needs to have a clear understanding of the features of subsequent therapeutic and preventive measures (organization of rational nutrition and motor regimen, prevention and treatment of residual pulmonary hypertension, infective endocarditis, circulatory failure, heart rhythm disturbances and conduction disturbances, thromboembolic complications, etc.) Moreover, since the number of patients who have reached child-bearing age has increased, and the probability of hereditary transmission of the pathological gene increases, which in turn, increases the possibility of having children with CHD, and this should also be taken into account by the pediatric cardiologist when diagnosing the expected CHD early [3].

The success of the treatment of patients with heart and blood vessels depends largely on how quickly they are detected, sent to a specialized institution, they establish a topical diagnosis. This is influenced by the degree of pulmonary hypertension, the severity of circulatory failure, the choice of treatment method and the timing of surgical correction of the defect. A timely treatment trend is an early surgical correction of congenital heart defects, but it is often possible to delay the surgery until a later date, when the risk of an adverse outcome becomes less.

It should be noted that in diseases of the heart, including congenital heart disease, the liver is affected due to an acute or chronic increase in central venous pressure, as well as a decrease in cardiac output. The phenomena of stagnation, necrosis, fibrosis, less often cirrhosis, which may exist separately, but are often combined depending on the clinical situation, are usually observed. To refer to these disorders, a number of authors [4, 5] suggest the term «cardiogenic liver».

Speaking about the importance of hemodynamic disorders in the pathogenesis of liver damage in diseases of the heart, it should be emphasized that the need for oxygen in the liver is comparable to that of the brain and the heart, and hypoxia significantly impairs its functions.

In the clinical picture one of the factors of liver damage most often prevails: stagnation due to right ventricular failure; insufficiency of arterial perfusion of the liver, caused by left ventricular failure; signs of cirrhosis against the background of long-term stagnation [3, 5].

Any heart disease causing an increase in pressure in the right atrium leads to stagnation of blood in the liver. The most common causes are mitral malformations, tricuspid valve insufficiency, congenital heart disease (atrial septal defect, patent ductus arteriosus, tetralogy of Fallot, single ventricle of the heart), pulmonary heart in chronic respiratory failure or recurrent thrombosis of small pulmonary artery branches, constrictive pericarditis, myocardial infarction of the right ventricle, right atrial myxoma.

The dependence of the liver's blood supply on the functional state of the right heart chambers is determined by the topographic relationship between the right atrium and the hepatic veins, the liver is called the reservoir for congestive blood, the right atrial pressure gauge.

Increased central venous pressure is transmitted to the hepatic veins and prevents blood flow to the central part of the lobule. Slowing blood circulation increases blood overflow in the central veins, the central part of the lobules. The developing central portal hypertension has mainly mechanical origin, hypoxia joins it. Localized central hypoxia causes atrophy and in some cases necrosis of hepatocytes. Cell death leads to collapse and condensation of the endoplasmic reticulum, active necrosis stimulates the formation of collagen, causes vein sclerosis. Further, the development of connective tissue leads to the displacement of the central veins to the portal site. Connective tissue bands connect the central veins of the adjacent lobules, and the architectonics of the liver is disturbed [5].

Macroscopically, the liver with heart failure is enlarged, dark red, full-blooded, it is rarely nodular. Expanded, distended veins protrude on the cut surface, the liver has the appearance of nutmeg (centrolobular red areas of stagnation and yellow rest of the lobules). Microscopically observed expansion of the central veins and sinusoids containing red blood cells, in some cases, the centers of the hepatic lobules have the appearance of «blood lakes». The trabecular structure is erased in the central areas, atrophy of hepatocytes develops, balloon degeneration, and as the process progresses, centrolobular focal necrosis is detected. Lipofuscin pigment in the form of tender or coarse clusters of golden yellow or brown color is contained in the center of hepatocytes [4, 5].

Both functional and morphological disorders of the liver can occur with a decrease in the arterial blood supply. The cause of such violations may be acute left ventricular failure or prolonged collapse, they are designated as ischemic hepatitis. As etiological factors, acute myocardial infarction, complicated by cardiogenic shock, arrhythmogenic collapses, postresuscitation conditions, septic, hypovolemic shock should be singled out.

With a decrease in perfusion pressure in the liver, sufficient oxygen saturation of the blood is observed only in the periportal zones and drops rapidly when approaching the central part of the lobule, which is most sensitive to metabolic damage. Severe hypoxia of centrolobular hepatic cells leads to the development of necrosis and, in some cases, an infarction [5].

According to various authors, the incidence of cirrhosis with congestive liver varies from 0,7 to 6,9% [3-5]. Most often it is detected on the background of long-term stagnation in the liver with tricuspid valve insufficiency or constrictive pericarditis. In addition to chronic stagnation, insufficient perfusion with the formation of centrolobular necrosis in the liver, long-term drug therapy, and protein-vitamin deficiency can be noted. Ultrasound examination (ultrasound) reveals, along with the characteristic signs of portal hypertension, the expansion of the lumen of the inferior vena cava. During the morphological study, in addition to the changes inherent in stagnation, periportal fibrosis, regenerate nodes, and reconstruction of lobular architectonics are revealed.

In the medical literature there are very few reports on the state of the liver, cholestatic disorders in children with congenital heart disease. Most publications concern Alagille syndrome.

TT. Gordon-Walker et al. [1] report on the development of cirrhosis and hepatocellular carcinoma in patients with CHD: single ventricle of the heart that underwent a radical correction of Fontan. The reason for the development of these conditions are hemodynamic changes associated with an increase in central venous pressure and a decrease in cardiac output. Heart-liver transplantation performed in the long term can help such patients.

In the study AM. Fattouh et al. [6], held at the Cairo University Children's Hospital, Egypt, reported the observation of 139 children aged 1 day to 7 months with various causes of cholestatic disorders. Of these, biliary atresia was diagnosed in 28% of patients, Alagille syndrome - in 11,5% of children. All patients underwent echocardiography. CHD were detected in 39,5% of patients. Shunting lesions were diagnosed in 43,6% of children, stenosis of the pulmonary artery in 32,7% of patients, combined defects in 16,4% of patients. 5,5% of children had an abnormal location of the heart. At the same time, CHD in patients with biliary atresia was detected in 35,9% of cases, in patients with Alagille syndrome in 93,7% of cases. The authors note that the majority of CHD in infants were asymptomatic.

G. Catli et al. [7] report a 40-day male infant with neonatal diabetes mellitus with atrial septal defect, pulmonic stenosis, and patent ductus arteriosus. The exocrine function of the pancreas was not impaired. In addition, the patient had transient idiopathic neonatal cholestasis and episodes of hypoglycemia not associated with insulin therapy. A genetic examination revealed a mutation of the GATA6 gene de novo.

H. Arnell, B. Fischler [8] examined 206 newborns with diagnosed Down syndrome, born between January 2005 and September 2011 in Stockholm, Sweden. CHD were detected in 47% of patients, congenital anomalies of the gastrointestinal tract in 11,2% of patients, neonatal cholestasis in 3,9% of children, and bone marrow diseases in 3,4% of patients. In addition, the authors concluded that neonatal cholestasis was more common in newborns with lesions of the gastrointestinal tract, CHD and bone marrow diseases.

Phenomena of cholestasis were severe in 3 patients (all of them had diseases of the bone marrow), characterized by liver failure and death in 2 cases. In 5 patients, cholestasis was transient.

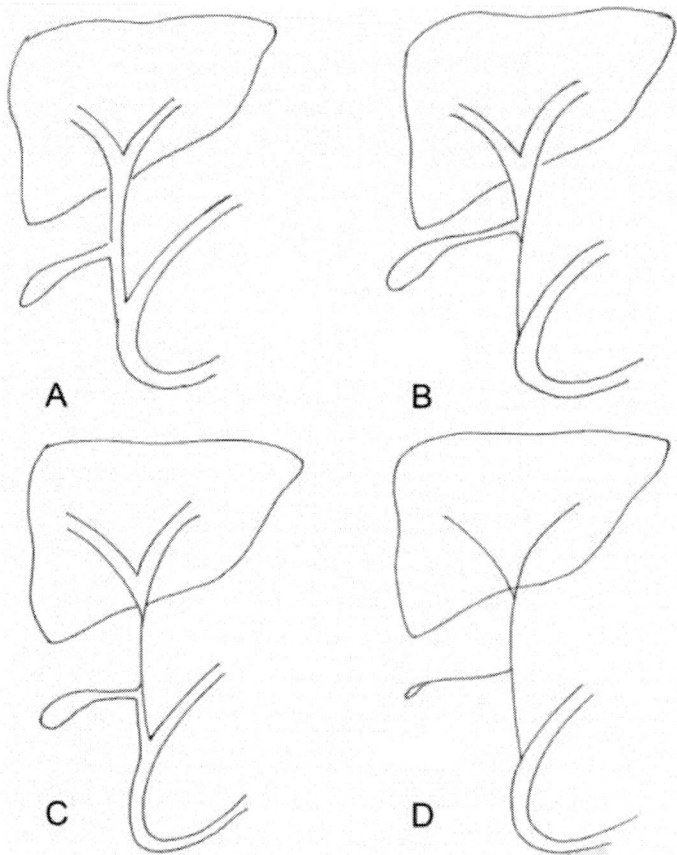

Picture 1. Classification of biliary atresia depending on the degree of involvement of the bile ducts.
A. Normal option.
B. Type 1; atresia of the common bile duct.
C. Type 2; atresia of the common hepatic duct.
D. Type 3; atresia of all extrahepatic bile ducts.

Among the causes of neonatal cholestasis, arteriohepatic dysplasia (Alagille syndrome) ranks second, occurring at a frequency of 1:70 000 newborns [9, 10]. The syndrome is characterized by an insufficient number or small diameter of the intrahepatic bile ducts, which remove bile from the liver (see Picture 1). Alagille syndrome includes a combination of at least three of the five main symptoms: chronic cholestasis, cardiovascular defects, spinal anomalies, eye defects, and characteristic craniofacial signs.

The syndrome was first described by the French pediatrician Daniel Alagille in 1975 as a disease with a typical combination of five signs: cholestasis, facial dysmorphism, incompetence of the bodies of predominantly thoracic vertebrae with a characteristic pattern of «butterfly» on the radiograph, pulmonic stenosis and/or its branches and other heart defects, ophthalmic abnormalities – posterior embryotoxon (congenital defect of the cornea), pigmentary retinopathy.

Alagille syndrome is inherited in an autosomal dominant manner. The gene defect is associated with a partial deletion of the short arm of the 20th chromosome [20p11-12], where the JAG1 gene is localized, as evidenced by molecular genetic research methods [10, 11].

The disease is characterized by an insufficient number or small diameter of the intrahepatic bile ducts, which complicates the outflow of bile and contributes to the accumulation of its components in the liver cells. The increased content of bile components in the blood plasma contributes to the appearance of painful pruritus. Insufficient flow of bile into the intestine leads to disruption of digestive processes. Malabsorption leads to delayed development and slow growth. Such patients often have broken bones, problems with vision, blood clotting, memory and learning. Characterized by delayed sexual development. Phenomena of cholestasis develop in the first 3 months of life and are characterized by jaundice with a greenish tinge, an increase in the size of the liver, an unstable Acholia of the chair, a dark urine color. The liver enlarges more due to the left lobe, which is smooth, painless, with a rounded edge, and its consistency is normal or moderately dense. The spleen is often enlarged. In Alagill's syndrome, fatty accumulations, called xanthomas, can form under the skin (on the dorsum of the finger joints, on the palmar surface of the hands, on the back of the neck, in the groin, around the anus). They are caused by abnormally high levels of cholesterol in the blood and indicate the severity of the process and duration of cholestasis. Characteristic phenotypic features are revealed: a high, prominent forehead, deep-set eyes, a straight nose, protruding ears, a protruding chin. In patients with Alagille syndrome, changes in the kidney are revealed – cysts, hypoplasia, dystopia of the kidneys, stenosis of the renal artery, renal stone disease, doubling of the ureter, etc. [10, 12].

Specific therapy is not developed. The treatment is aimed at maintaining the functions of the affected organs and reducing the symptoms of the disease. To improve liver function, hepatoprotective drugs are used; to reduce jaundice and itching – preparations of ursodeoxycholic acid. In severe cases, liver transplantation is performed.

If atresia of the intrahepatic bile ducts is expressed slightly (only a small amount of bile ducts is missing), the prognosis is favorable and complications usually do not occur. In most cases, atresia is significant, which is unfavorable for prognosis; during the first years of life, cirrhosis of the liver develops - patients die from liver failure. Liver transplantation allows patients to prolong life, but in the case of a combination with a severe heart defect, its conduction causes great doubts [12, 13].

EV. Omelchenko et al. [13] describe an 11-month-old boy with Alagille syndrome, characterized by intrahepatic cholestasis with the development of secondary biliary cirrhosis with hepatic insufficiency, CHD (secondary atrial septal defect), changes in the musculoskeletal system (facial dysmorphia, lumbar anomalies) – sacral junction (L6 lumbarization, spina bifida L6), agendus of the coccyx), physical development lag. The child's illness has been fatal due to end-stage liver failure and the inability to perform a liver transplant.

Girl, 16 years old, with Alagille syndrome was also observed in our department of pediatric cardiac surgery and rehabilitation of the Institute of Emergency and Reconstructive Surgery named after VC. Husak of Donetsk [12]. Alagille syndrome is characterized by hypoplasia of the intrahepatic bile ducts, the CHD (peripheral pulmonary artery stenosis), changes of the musculoskeletal system (facial dysmorphia, scoliosis of the thoracic and lumbar spine, low back pain lumbar arthralgia), a feature of the structure of the organ of vision (rear embryotoxon) lag in physical and sexual development. A genetic screening performed in Zurich, Switzerland, revealed a mutation of the JAG1 gene de novo.

MC. Digilio et al. [14] report on a patient with Alagille syndrome and tetralogy of Fallot. Alagille syndrome was characterized by moderate liver involvement in the form of a small increase in the level of aminotransferases and direct bilirubin in the blood. In addition, there were facial abnormalities, delayed speech development with a nasal voice, learning difficulties. A genetic examination revealed a mutation of the JAG1 gene and a deletion of 22q11.2. These molecular data confirm the cumulative effect of multiple genetic defects in the etiology of human malformations.

ML. Robert et al. [15] report a 4-year-old patient with Alagille syndrome associated with hypoplastic left heart syndrome. The boy was born on the 37th week of pregnancy weighing 1885g. After birth, he was diagnosed hypoplastic left heart syndrome, about which the Norwood procedure was performed. In the future, the child was lagging behind in physical and neuropsychic development, paying attention to facial dysmorphism. A genetic examination revealed a deletion of 20p12.2-p12.3. In addition, an in-depth study found posterior embryotoxon and vertebrae in the form of a «butterfly». Liver function tests remained normal.

RC. Bauer et al. [16] emphasize the need for an in-depth examination, including a genetic study, of patients with right-sided heart disease (tetralogy of Fallot, pulmonic stenosis) for possible Alagille syndrome.

RD. Mainwaring et al. [17], MC. Monge et al. [18] reported good results of surgical correction of CHD in patients with Alagille syndrome. However, the long-term prognosis is determined by the polyorganism of the lesion with this syndrome.

JJ. Hofmann et al. [19] in experimental work demonstrate that endothelial deletion of JAG1 in mice leads to the development of cardiovascular abnormalities resembling defects in Alagille syndrome. In mutant mice, right ventricular hypertrophy, ventricular septal defect, coronary anomalies, and valve defects were detected. In addition, in adult mutant mice, heart valve calcification was detected. The authors note that the endothelium is responsible for a wide range of cardiac phenotypes associated with Alagille syndrome, and demonstrate the important role of JAG1 in valve morphogenesis.

The purpose of our research was to study the state of the liver in children with congenital heart disease.

Under the supervision there were 45 children with CHD who were hospitalized in the Department of Pediatric Cardiology and Cardiac Surgery of the Institute of Emergency and Reconstructive Surgery named after VC. Gusak, Donetsk, from September to December 2018. The age of the surveyed ranged from 2 months to 17 years. Boys observed 28 people (62,2%), girls – 17 people (37,8%). All patients underwent an in-depth examination: blood count, urinalysis, blood biochemical parameters (bilirubin, transaminases, proteinogram, prothrombin index), TORCH markers, electrocardiogram, echocardiography, ultrasound of the liver and gall bladder, according to the indications genetics consultation.

The results of our study indicate that CHD are represented by: a ventricular septal defect in 12 (26,7%) people, a secondary atrial septal defect in 11 (24,4%) people, double discharge of the main vessels from the right ventricle – in 7 (15,6%) people, common atrioventricular canal – in 7 (15,6%) people, tetralogy of Fallot – in 5 (11,1%) people, Ebstein's anomaly – in 1 (2,2%) people, coarctation of the aorta – in 1 (2,2%) persons, stenosis of the aortic mouth – in 1 (2,2%) persons. Combined CHD were diagnosed in 8 (17,8%) children. Abnormal location of the heart in combination with CHD was observed in 1 (2,2%) patient.

All patients had signs of chronic heart failure (CHF). Of these, CHF 1, according to the classification of ND. Strazhesko, VH. Vasilenko [3], registered in 17 (37,8%) patients, CHF 2a – in 24 (53,3%) patients, CHF 2b – in 4 (8,9%) children.

The following concomitant pathologies in children were: Down syndrome – in 8 (17,8%) people, Shereshevsky-Turner syndrome – in 1 (2,2%) people, Arnold-Chiari anomaly – in 1 (2.2%) people, subclinical hypothyroidism – in 3 (6,7%) people. Rachitis was diagnosed in 17 (37,8%) patients, timomegaly in 4 (8,9%) children, delayed physical development in 8 (17,8%) patients, iron deficiency anemia in 10 (22,2%) children, atopic dermatitis – in 3 (6,7%) patients, cryptorchidism – in 2 (4,4%) patients.

In addition, cardiac rhythm and conduction disorders were detected in the examined patients. So, extrasystole was registered in 10 (22,2%) children, blockade of the right bundle branch block – in 2 (4,4%) patients, WPW phenomenon – in 1 (2,2%) patient, congenital heart block – in 1 (2,2%) patient.

Complaints of nausea, feeling of heaviness while eating, pain in the right hypochondrium presented to 9 (20,0%) children. An objective examination showed an increase and hardening of the liver in 34 (75,6%) patients, an increase in the spleen – in 6 (13,3%) children. Ascites and edema in the lower limbs were observed in 4 (8,9%) patients.

With additional examination, increases in the level of aminotransferases were not registered in any case. Reduction in the level of albumin, prothrombin index in the blood was also not observed in the examined patients. Hyperbilirubinemia due to the indirect fraction was observed in 3 (6,7%) patients. Immunological examination revealed an association with Epstein-Barr virus – in 5 (11,1%) children, herpes simplex virus ½ type – in 4 (8.9%) patients, and with AIDS virus – in 1 (2,2%) patient. With ultrasound, signs of hepatosplenomegaly as a manifestation of portal hypertension syndrome were observed in 34 (75,6%) patients, tortuosity and deformity of the gallbladder – in 7 (15,6%) children.

Thus, the survey results indicate that ¾ children with CHD and CHF had hepatosplenomegaly. An enlarged liver in most cases was the result of hemodynamic disorders and venous congestion of the blood in it.

REFERENCES

[1] Gordon-Walker, TT; Bove, K; Veldtman, G. Fontan-associated liver disease: A review. *J Cardiol.*, 2019, Mar 27. pii: S0914-5087(19)30059-0. doi: 10.1016/j.jjcc.2019.02.016. [Epub ahead of print] Review.

[2] Cangussú, LR; Lopes, MR; Barbosa, RHA. The importance of the early diagnosis of aorta coarctation. *Rev Assoc Med Bras*, (1992), 2019 Feb, 65(2), 240-245. doi: 10.1590/1806-9282.65.2.240.

[3] Mutafian, OA. Congenital heart diseases in children. *SPb.: Nevsky Dialect*, 2002.
[4] Perederiy, VG; Tkach, SM. Practical Gastroenterology: a manual for physicians. *Vinnitsa*, 2011.
[5] Podymova, SD. Diseases of the liver. Manual for doctors. M.: *Medicine*, 1998.
[6] Fattouh, AM; Mogahed, EA; Abdel Hamid, N; Sobhy, R; Saber, N; El-Karaksy, H. The prevalence of congenital heart defects in infants with cholestatic disorders of infancy: a single-centre study. *Arch. Dis. Child.*, 2016, 15.
[7] Catli, G; Abaci, A; Flanagan, SE; De Franko, E; Ellard, S; Hattersley, A; et al. A novel GATA6 mutation leading to congenital heart defects and permanent neonatal diabetes: a case report. *Diabetes Metab.*, 2013, 39(4), 370-4.
[8] Arnell, H; Fischler, B. Population-based study of incidence and clinical outcome of neonatal cholestasis in patients with Down syndrome. *J. Pediatr.*, 2012, 161(5), 899-902.
[9] Berniczei-Royko, A; Chalas, R; Mitura, I; Nagy, K; Prussak, E. Medical and dental management of Alagille syndrome: a review. *Med. Sci. Monit.*, 2014, 24(20), 476-80.
[10] Turnpenny, PD; Ellard, S. Alagille syndrome: pathogenesis, diagnosis and management. *Eur. J. Hum. Genet.*, 2012, 20(3), 251-7.
[11] Nemir, M; Pedrazzini, T. Functional role of Notch signaling in the developing and postnatal heart. *J. Mol. Cell. Cardiol.*, 2008, 45(4), 495-504.
[12] Nagornaya, NV; Bordyugova, EV; Dubovaya, AV; Smirnova, TV. Alagille Syndrome. *Health child.*, 2008, 4 (13).
[13] Omelchenko, EV; Yermolaev, MN; Senatorova, AS; Shipko, AF; Omelchenko-Selyukova, AV; Yermolaeva, MM; et al. Clinical case of Alagille syndrome. *Health child.*, 2015, 62, 128-32.
[14] Digilio, MC; Luca, AD; Lepri, F; Guida, V; Dentici, ML; Angioni, A; et al. JAG1 mutation in a patient with deletion 22q11.2 syndrome and tetralogy of Fallot. *Am. J. Med. Genet. A.*, 2013, 161A(12), 3133-6.

[15] Robert, ML; Lopez, T; Crolla, J; Huang, S; Owen, C; Burvill-Holmes, L; et al. Alagille syndrome with deletion 20p12.2-p12.3 and hypoplastic left heart. *Clin. Dysmorphol.*, 2007, 16(4), 241-6.

[16] Bauer, RC; Laney, AO; Smith, R; Gerfen, J; Morrissette, JJ; Woyciechowsky, S; et al. Jagged1 (JAG1) mutations in patients with tetralogy of Fallot or pulmonic stenosis. *Hum. Mutat.*, 2010, 31(5), 594-601.

[17] Mainwaring, RD; Sheikh, AY; Punn, R; Reddy, VM; Hanley, FL. Surgical outcomes for patients with pulmonary atresia/major aortopulmonary collaterals and Alagille syndrome. *Eur. J. Cardiothorac. Surg.*, 2012, 42(2), 235-40.

[18] Monge, MC; Mainwaring, RD; Sheikh, AY; Punn, R; Reddy, VM; Hanley, FL. Surgical reconstruction of peripheral pulmonary artery stenosis in Williams and Alagille syndromes. *J. Thorac. Cardiovasc. Surg.*, 2013, 145(2), 476-81.

[19] Hofmann, JJ; Briot, A; Ensico, J; Zovein, AC; Ren, S; Zhang, ZW; et al. Endothelial deletion of murine Jag1 leads to valve calcification and congenital heart defects associated with Alagille syndrome. *Development*. 2012, 139(23), 4449-60.

BIOGRAPHICAL SKETCH

Name: Lymarenko Maryna

Affiliation: Donetsk National Medical University named after M. Gorky

Education: higher

Business Address: Illich Avenue, 16, Donetsk, Ukraine

Research and Professional Experience: Candidate of Medical Sciences, Associate Professor

Professional Appointments: pediatric cardiology, pediatric gastroenterology, pediatric nephrology

Honors: certificates and gratitude of the Donetsk National Medical University named after M. Gorky

Publications from the Last 3 Years:

[1] Lymarenko, MP. Clinical observation of a combination of congenital heart disease and the reverse location of internal organs. Proceedings of the XII International Congress "Cardiostim". St. Petersburg., 2016, 196.
[2] Lymarenko, MP; Aladyina, DA; Sosna, VV. Stenosis of the aortic mouth: a review of literature and personal observation. University Hospital., 2016, 12(1), 106-110.
[3] Lymarenko, MP. Fermentopathy as the cause of atopic dermatitis in children. Collection of scientific and practical. *Works "Health Bulletin".*, 2016, 1(2), 302-306.
[4] Lymarenko, MP; Parshinova, AE. Klippel-Feil syndrome: a review of the literature and its own clinical observation. *Bulletin of Emergency and Reconstructive Surgery.*, 2018, 3(2), 154-157.
[5] Pshenichnaya, EV; Limarenko, MP; Marchenko, EN; Kolomenskaya, SA; Shevtsova, EI. Clinical observation of paroxysmal night hemoglobinuria in a teenager. *Herald of emergency and restorative surgery.* 2018, 3(2), 192-197.

In: Congenital Heart Disease
Editor: Curtis Giguère

ISBN: 978-1-53616-674-3
© 2020 Nova Science Publishers, Inc.

Chapter 6

HIGH ALTITUDE AND CONGENITAL HEART DISEASE IN ANDEAN HIGHLANDS POPULATIONS: THE CASE OF ECUADOR

Fabricio González-Andrade[1,2], Stephanie Michelena[1,4], Daniel Echeverría Espinosa[1,3] and Gabriela Aguinaga Romero[1]

[1]Universidad Central del Ecuador, Facultad de Ciencias Médicas, Unidad de Medicina Traslacional, Quito, Ecuador
[2]Universidad San Francisco de Quito USFQ, Colegio Ciencias de la Salud, Quito, Ecuador
[3]Hospital Baca Ortiz (HBO), Quito, Ecuador
[4]School of Biomedical Science, University of Queensland, St Lucia QLD, Australia

ABSTRACT

It is estimated that there are around 83 million people living at high altitudes; over 2500 meters above sea level (masl) worldwide. Andean (highlands), Tibetan, and Ethiopian populations have lived under chronic hypoxia conditions for thousands of years. From those, groups who have been residing there for over a millennium in three high-altitude zones of the globe are the Sherpa and Ayurveda (Qinghai-Tibetan Plateau), the Kichwa and Aymara highlanders (Andean Altiplano), and the Ethiopian Amhara and Oromo highlanders (the Semien Plateau in Ethiopia). For them, the adaptive and maladaptive changes have occurred at the genomic and physiological levels. In Ecuador, for example, most of the capital cities are located at altitudes above 2500 masl.

High-altitude hypoxia presents numerous challenges to human health, survival, and reproduction due to the decreased oxygen availability brought on by lowered barometric pressure at high elevations. Changes in pulmonary function, arterial oxygen saturation (SaO_2) hemoglobin concentration, and maternal physiology during pregnancy among others have permitted high-altitude natives to thrive in the harsh conditions. Most common adaptative changes involves ventilation rates, hypoxic ventilatory response, elevated arterial oxygen saturation, elevated hemoglobin concentration, and elevated birth weight.

Despite these adaptations, it seems that some diseases are more commonly observed within these populations. For instance, the prevalence of Congenital Heart Disease (CHD) in newborns at high altitude is about 20 times higher than at low altitude. High altitude is an environmental risk factor for CHD, especially patent ductus arteriosus (PDA). By 18 months of age, about 60% of left to right shunts remain unclosed. Atrial Septal Defect (ASD), Ventricular Septal Defect (VSD) and Left Ventricular Outflow tract obstruction LVOTO are show frequently at high altitude.

Researchers have tried to explain the role of high altitude on CHD for over 60 years, describing different mechanisms, including embryonic tissue hypoxia. The increase frequency of CHD at high altitudes clearly suggest a leading role for environmental mechanisms mediated by low atmospheric pressure and the persistence of pulmonary hypertension after birth. Screening newborn children for CHD) mostly focus on critical CHD using pulse oximetry.

This is a review of high altitude adaptation, and its effects on CHD focused in the Andean region, and in Ecuador as a study case.

Keywords: congenital heart disease, high altitude, chronic adaptation, Andean populations, Native Americans, Ecuador

INTRODUCTION

Linking human evolutionary history with the current knowledge in biology and genetics has allowed us to understand human evolution. One of the few environments that can provide natural experimental settings at which humans have been evolving is at high-altitude regions, 2500 meters above sea level (masl) (Beall 2000). Moreover, only 2% of the world's population thrive at these high-altitude regions, representing over 140 million people (Hurtado et al. 2012). Biological adaptability has facilitated us the occupation of this type of environments with a variety of unique features such as high UV radiation, limited-diet and low-temperature (Beall 2007).

High altitude locations are characterized by unique environmental factors, one of these is the low air compressibility. Even though the amount of oxygen remains constant (20.93%) in both at high and low altitudes, the number of gaseous molecules per unit volume is greater at low altitude than at high altitude, hence, the barometric pressure, which depends on the molecular concentration of the air, has an inversely proportional relationship with the altitude at which it is measured. This particular pressure follows a non-linear trend (Brown and Grocott 2013; Frisancho 2013). For example, at sea level, barometric pressure is 760 mm Hg and the partial pressure of oxygen (pO2) is 159 mm Hg. Meanwhile, at 3,500 masl the barometric pressure is reduced to 493 mm Hg and the pO2 is 103 mm Hg, meaning that oxygen has about 35% less pressure at high altitude than at sea level.

In other terms, a breath of air at 4,000 meters elevation contains roughly 60% of the oxygen molecules that it has at sea level. Therefore, people living in this environment are exposed to a decrease in oxygen per inspired air which results in less oxygen available to be diffused into the bloodstream and ultimately, less oxygen for energy production in cells. This represents a limitation to eukaryotic organisms, because all of them rely on oxygen for efficient adenosine triphosphate (ATP) production, necessary for proper tissue development, homeostasis, and function (Krock, Skuli, and Simon 2011). This limitation exists, as humans are not capable of storing oxygen, due to the violent reactive nature of this element with other molecules in the body. For this reason, is essential that oxygen is supplied steadily to the mitochondria and to the cell and tissues that require oxygen for enzymatic reactions (Beall 2007).

Proper tissue oxygenation relies on the balance between oxygen supply and the demand generated by metabolic reactions on tissues. People living at high altitudes face lower oxygen availability for gas exchange in the lungs which results in an impaired tissue oxygenation. Due to the lower amount of oxygen delivered to the cells, by the respiratory, hematological and cardiovascular systems, a physiological condition called hypoxia often develops (Frisancho 2013). Some of the implications of decreased oxygen are headaches, nausea and dizziness. As a result of this, populations have endured this conditions for years and have developed physiological and genetical adaptations for this environment (Gonzales, Alarcón-Yaquetto, and Zevallos-Concha 2016). For example, the Qinghai-Tibetan Plateau, the Andean and the Ethiopian highlanders exhibit unique circulatory, respiratory, and hematological adaptations. They also display physiological differences within one another (Bigham et al. 2013). In this chapter, the physiological changes as well as the differences between these high-altitude living groups will be summarized. The fascinating genetic mechanisms that allow them to adapt to the harsh conditions at more than 2500 masl will also be outlined.

PHYSIOLOGICAL ADAPTATIONS

Physiological changes at high altitude can occur at short term (acute adaptation from one to three months) and long term (chronic adaptation for more than seven years). Some changes that have occurred over a number of generations as a result of natural selection for living in a hypobaric hypoxic environment, are often denoted under a process called acclimatization (Grocott, Montgomery, and Vercueil 2007). This enhances survival and performance due to oxygen delivery to the cells is improved through adjustments in the cardiovascular, respiratory and hematologic systems (Paralikar and Paralikar 2010). Adjustments are necessary in an environment where humidity, air density and temperature have decreased considerably. These factors may contribute to airway reactivity, ventilatory changes, insensible water losses, and alterations in pulmonary hemodynamics (Stream, Luks, and Grissom 2009). The physiological responses to chronic cold exposure, also known as cold acclimation/

acclimatization, are also presented. Three primary patterns of cold acclimatization have been observed, a) habituation, b) metabolic adjustment, and c) insulative adjustment.

Andean and Tibetan highlanders exhibit a standard low-altitude range of oxygen delivery from minimal to maximal. They also have a different normal basal metabolic rate and maximal oxygen uptake expected for their sex, age, and body weight (Picón-Reátegui 1961). These differences suggest that their functional adaptations do not require an increase on basal oxygen. A study of people living at 3,900 masl showed that the maximum oxygen consumption was 47 ml/O_2 per kilogram, and 46 ml/O_2 per kilogram for Andeans and Tibetans respectively. These values are similar for untrained men at sea level and 10% to 20% higher for low altitude natives residing at the same altitudes. This suggests that the mechanism of aerobic potential is unchanged between high and low altitude populations. Even though both populations have similar functional endpoint, measurements of oxygen delivery along the transport cascade are different (Beall 2007).

One of the physiological adaptations within the respiratory system includes pulmonary ventilation. Exposure to hypoxia stimulates the carotid and aortic body and peripheral chemoreceptors to signal the central respiratory center in the medulla to increase ventilation, thus lowering alveolar carbon dioxide improving oxygen delivery (Paralikar and Paralikar 2010). Hyperventilation decreases the partial pressure of carbon dioxide (PCO_2) at the alveoli, which increases pulmonary vascular resistance and pulmonary artery pressure (PAP), 12 ± 2.2 mm Hg at sea level to 28 ± 10.5 mm Hg at high altitude (Penaloza and Arias-Stella 2007). Due to the decrease in PCO_2 excess, a condition called alkalosis (blood pH >7.4) can occur. The human body reacts by rapidly removing bicarbonates from the blood (Frisancho 2013). High levels of PAP results in pulmonary hypertension and is both accompanied and caused by pulmonary vascular remodeling. The pulmonary vascular wall consists of three layers: adventitia, media and intima, whose cellular components are fibroblasts, smooth muscle cells (SMC) and endothelial cells (EC), respectively. Hypoxia is able to increase cell proliferation by the inhibition of antimitogenic factors and by increasing the production of different mitogenic stimuli and inflammatory mediators from SMC, fibroblasts, EC and platelets (Pak et al. 2007).

Consequently, on Andean populations the hypobaric condition appears to blunt the hypoxic ventilatory response (HVR) that leads to hypoventilation compared to sea level populations. This hypoventilation results in low arterial oxygen pressure that in turn increases erythropoiesis, increasing hematocrit levels that may aid oxygen transport (Chiodi 1957). A study on high altitude natives at 3900 masl reported resting ventilation of 15 liters/min for Tibetans whereas for Andeans had 10.5 liters/min (Beall 2007). Therefore, it can be inferred that these physiological changes might be unique to Tibetans. Additionally, alveoli hypoxia often causes pulmonary vasoconstriction (HPV) to divert blood into better-oxygenated lung segments, optimizing ventilation/perfusion matching and systemic oxygen delivery (Dunham-Snary et al. 2017). This vasoconstriction is caused by the inhibition of potassium channels that depolarize the pulmonary artery smooth muscle cells increasing cytosolic calcium resulting in vasoconstriction.

Other adaptations involve the diffusion capacity and the lung volume. The oxygen pulmonary diffusing capacity of lowland natives remains constant at both high altitudes and sea level (Frisancho 2013). In contrast, Andean populations have an increased efficiency of oxygen transfer as a result of a greater total lung capacity and residual volume, volume of air remaining in lungs after maximum expiration. These characteristics give rise to the barrel-chest Andean morphology with lung volume expansion and increased lung growth which is common in high-altitude residents (Julian and Moore 2019a).

The hematopoietic response is another important acclimatization factor. Hemoglobin is a protein in red blood cells (RBC) that carries oxygen from the lungs to the tissues. Hemoglobin concentration is influenced by many factors, one of them is the presence of erythropoietin, a protein that causes differentiation of the precursors that will become hemoglobin-containing RBC. As a response to hypoxia at high altitudes plasma volume decreases, while erythropoiesis increase resulting in augmentation of total hemoglobin and RBC mass (Vargas 2014). Thus, highland natives have RBC counts from five to eight million compared to four million at low altitudes. Hemoglobin also increases from 12-16 g/100ml at sea level to 17 -20 g/100 ml at high altitudes (Merino 2009). A study of residents of Potosi in Bolivia living at 4000 masl suggested that hematocrit levels range from 45% to 61% in men and 41% to 56% in women while normal values at sea levels are 45 to 52% in men and 37 to 48% in women (Vásquez and Villena 2002).

On the other hand, the affinity of oxygen for hemoglobin quantified is P_{50}, the arterial oxygen tension at which hemoglobin is 50% saturated with oxygen. This affinity is determined by the hemoglobin structure and is influenced by CO_2, H^+ and temperature. Another hematopoietic response can be observed by analyzing the sigmoidal relationship between oxygen partial pressure and oxygen saturation of hemoglobin. This shifts to the left during initial exposure to hypoxia where hyperventilation and alkalosis are present, however, it is then compensated by a 2,3-diphosphoglycerate increase correcting the shift rightward (Jansen et al. 2007; Brown and Grocott 2013). The product of hemoglobin concentration and oxygen saturation is known as hemoglobin oxygen saturation, which is found to higher on the Andean highlanders (22.3ml/100mL) compared to sea level populations (20ml/100mL) (Jansen and Basnyat 2011; Jansen et al. 2007).

In regard to oxygen and blood distribution which can be observed from the fact that the capacity of highlanders to perform physical work is superior compared to lowlanders who are sojourning those elevations. Levels of cardiac output at a given workload are comparable between acclimatized newcomers and Andean permanent inhabitants, while at maximal exercise values in both groups are lower compared to sea level (Vogel, Hartley, and Cruz 1974). An active suppression by central nervous system, an increased afterload due to arterial pressure and decreased filling has been suggested as a possible explanation. However, the actual reasons for this reduction in cardiac output remains unknown (Julian and Moore 2019b).

On another topic, regional blood flow determines oxygen distribution. During exercise, blood flow to the periphery and fractional oxygen extraction are decreased in Andean inhabitants when compared with acclimatized lowlanders. This is due to blood being diverted to other tissues (Lundby et al. 2006). As an example, high altitude Andean inhabitants show

18% lower resting middle cerebral flow velocities than at low altitude populations, suggesting that one if not all factors in charge on the regulation brain blood flow, hematocrit, arterial oxygen saturation, nitric oxide (NO) availability and brain metabolism might be involved in the chronic adaptation process (Jansen and Basnyat 2011). For this, brain blood flow was measured by blood flow velocity through internal carotid, vertebral and middle cerebral arteries. Considerations should be taken as blood flow also depends on vessel diameter and cross-sectional area (Julian and Moore 2019b). Thus, oxygen distribution is another factor that distinguish Andean population from other high-altitude communities.

Furthermore, as everything in the body, blood flow is autoregulated. Cerebral autoregulation (CA) is the capacity of the brain to maintain blood supply constant. This Mechanism protects the brain from ischemia at low arterial pressure, prevents the disruption of the blood-brain barrier and the formation of brain edema at high arterial pressure. Disturbed CA is usually reported in traumatic brain injury, ischemic stroke, malignant hypertension and after cardiac arrest. Besides this, it has also been reported in the Sherpa individuals, community living above 4000 masl. Causality theories includes first, vasodilation of the cerebral vessels resulting on increased cerebral blood flow and second, a lack of vessels contractility. This in turn enhances vasodilator activity, such as the release of NO; or inhibition of vasoconstrictors, such as endothelin-1 (Jansen et al. 2007). During hypoxia red blood cells are capable to release NO even far from their location of formation which accounts for hypoxia-induced vasodilatation. In this respect, exhalation of NO by Tibetan and Andean populations living at 4,200 masl is higher compared to sea-level subjects (Beall, Laskowski, and Erzurum 2012).

Highlanders also show anatomical and physiological characteristics on their cardiovascular system that has allowed them to adapt to high-altitude chronic hypoxia. Coronary flow at high altitude is on average 49mL/min/100g whereas at sea level is 71.7mL/min/100g (Moret 1971). Even though the decrease in flow is not compensated by the increased hematocrit, there is no sign of insufficient oxygenation of the myocardium as oxygen extraction by the heart is enhanced (Hurtado et al. 2012).

Interestingly, a study demonstrates that subjects living at high altitude have increased number of branches and peripheral vessels in the coronary vasculature compared with those found in people who live at sea level (Arias and Topilsky 1971).

In addition, oxygen delivery is used to convert food into chemical energy by adenosine triphosphate (ATP) synthesis in the mitochondria. Because ATP production efficiency depends strongly on the fuel source, during chronic hypoxia, a response from the myocardium is to metabolize glucose over free fatty acid or lipids. The main reason for this is that carbohydrate oxidation yields 25 to 50% more ATP per mole of oxygen than fat oxidation. In fact, during glycogen breakdown the energy expended in their synthesis is almost entirely recovered. In contrast, in the hydrolysis of triacylglycerol to fatty acids the ATP that was consumed is not recovered (Holden et al. 1995) It was found that Quechua male population relies on carbohydrate metabolism for heart functioning with 50-60% more ATP produced per mole of oxygen compared with lowlanders, this increased oxygen efficiency in the heart suggests a biochemical adaptation for hypoxia (Holden et al. 1995).

Residences at high altitude also alter glucose metabolism. Glucose uptake is increased, and glucose tolerance is improved, thus venous glucose levels are lower at high altitude (Woolcott, Ader, and Bergman 2015). From available data a median fasting plasma glucose concentration is 81.6 mg/dL for adult males living above 3000 m, whereas in residents from low altitude the estimated value was 91.2 mg/dL. Likewise, an inverse association between altitude and fasting glycemia has been shown, 85mg/dL at 1000 masl, 83mg/dL between 1000 to 2999 masl and 78.8mg/dL at 3000 masl (Pajuelo, Sánchez, and Arbañil 2010). This evidence suggests a better glycemic control at higher altitude. However, there are few studies that have reported no difference in fasting glycemia between highlanders and lowlanders. Thus, further research needs to be done for concluding evidence.

Furthermore, the mechanism behind lower fasting glycemia at high altitudes is not fully understood. Glucose entry into the bloodstream depends on diet, peripheral glucose disposal and endogenous sources like the liver which in fact controls blood glucose concentration. During fasting, around

80% of blood glucose is supplied by the liver and 20% by the kidney (Gerich et al. 1963). For this reason, lower fasting glycemia among highlanders could be the result of a low glucose production in the liver (Woolcott, Ader, and Bergman 2015). Another explanation for lower fasting glycemia involves the adipose tissue. Stored lipids breakdown in adipose tissue release fatty acids into the bloodstream. Fasting hyperglycemia is caused by elevated fatty acid levels which enhance gluconeogenesis and glycogenolysis (Staehr et al. 2003). Hence, lower fatty acids levels may explain the lower fasting glycemia. As a matter of fact, fatty acids values depend various factors such as the type of diet, lipolysis and fasting duration (Qaid and Abdelrahman 2016). More studies are needed in order to determine highlander's fatty acid levels.

Interestingly, evidence shows a lower prevalence of diabetes on high altitude communities. Some studies report a link between environmental factors, vitamin D and solar radiation, and diabetes (MITRI and PITTAS 2014). Solar ultraviolet (UV)-B radiation increases proportionally with altitude, approximately by 7% every kilometer. Thus, the possibility that the lower prevalence of diabetes at higher altitudes could be accounted for by solar radiation should be considered. Nevertheless, this later possibility seems to be unlikely because administration of vitamin D_2 in humans has failed to modify insulin sensitivity a key component in the pathogenesis of diabetes (Simha et al. 2016).

Hypoxia affect directly the kidneys, specially the systemic acid-base balance, neuroendocrine reflexes, ventilation and hemodynamics that in turn alter renal function and fluid balance (Swenson and Bärtsch 2013). In high-altitude residents, renal blood flow (RBF) and glomerular filtration rate (GFR) are decreased by 12%, renal plasma flow is decreased by 30 to 40% as a result of secondary polycythemia whereas filtration fraction increases by 39%. Besides this, kidney oxygen delivery, arteriovenous gradients, and consumption are maintained compared to sea-level values (Luks, Johnson, and Swenson 2008).

On the other hand, the mitochondria, itself, also play an important role during hypoxia at high altitude to maintain cellular homeostasis. One to two percent of molecular oxygen is converted to reactive oxygen species (ROS) due to electron leak from the electron transport chain. ROS, such as the superoxide radical (O_2^-), are molecules with unpaired electrons that are potentially toxic for the human body. For this reason, there is an antioxidant defend system which limits tissue damage (Jefferson et al. 2004). Literature also suggests that as hypoxia reduces oxygen availability there is a decrease on the generation of free radicals. Despite this, recent studies indicated an increased risk of oxidative stress at high altitudes due to ultraviolet light, diet and temperature. Thus, generating an increase of ROS (Murray and Horscroft 2016). When compared to lowlanders, 8-iso-PGF2alpha, plasma TBARS and glutathione, markers of ROS, are increased in high altitude Andean populations (Jefferson et al. 2004).

These physiological changes are not exclusive to cardiovascular and metabolic processes, they also occur in the skeletal muscle system. This is one of the major tissues of the body representing almost 40% of body weight. Skeletal muscle is composed of fibers with distinct contractile and metabolic properties. Type I fibers, or slow oxidative, are cells with high number of mitochondria, myoglobin and capillary density. Type IIX and IIB fibers, or fast glycolytic, have larger cross-sectional area with higher glycolytic machinery, and type IIA, or fast oxidative, exhibit an intermediate properties (Favier et al. 2015). Due to that more than 90% of the energy produced by muscle cells comes from the aerobic pathway, a reduction in oxygen availability would challenge skeletal muscle homeostasis. Skeletal muscle is capable to modify its size and adjust its metabolic and contractile properties to a variety of stimuli including mechanical strains and neuronal activity metabolic and hormonal influences, as well as environmental factors. Chronic exposure to high altitude has been shown to affect the structural, functional and metabolic profiles of skeletal muscle (Fluck 2006). Highlanders possess a greater number of capillaries as well as lower muscle fiber per cross-sectional area of muscle, when compared with lowlanders. Thus, increasing capillary density-to-muscle fiber ratio (Gilbert-Kawai et al. 2014). Additionally, literature indicates an increased on cytochrome *c* reductase activity (+78%) and myoglobin content (+16%) in biopsies of sartorius muscle of permanent high-altitude residents as compared to lowlanders. Conversely, there is a 25% decrease on muscle mitochondrial volume density compared with lowland populations (Hoppeler et al. 1990). Myoglobin is a protein that allows oxygen storage and diffusion in cardiac and skeletal muscle. This protein adjusts oxygen inflow efficiently and its consumption in skeletal muscles through links with the regulation of NO concentration. Therefore, it may serve a role in hypoxic adaptation. In fact, Andean living at high altitude have a higher concentration of myoglobin than those living at sea level (Reynafarje 1961).

Table 1. Summary of physiological changes

	Physiological adaptations	References
Respiratory	Blunt hypoxic ventilatory response	Chiodi 1957
	Normal maximal oxygen uptake	Picón-Reátegui 1961
	Normal basal metabolic rate	Picón-Reátegui 1961
	Increased diffusion capacity	Frisancho 2013
	Increased lung volume	Frisancho 2013; Julian and Moore 2019a
Circulatory	Increased hematocrit	Vásquez and Villena 2002
	Increased erythropoiesis	Vargas 2014; Merino 2009
Cardiac	Myocardium shows enhanced oxygen extraction	Hurtado 2012
	Reduced cardiac output	Vogel, Hartley, and Cruz 1974; Julian and Moore 2019b
	Decreased coronary blood flow	Moret 1971; Hurtado et al. 2012
	Physiological adaptations	References
Muscular	Increased capillary number	Favier et al. 2015; Gilbert-Kawai et al. 2014
	Reduced mitochodrial volume density	Favier et al. 2015; Hoppeler et al. 1990
	Increased myoglobin content	Reynafarje 1961
	Increased cytochrome C reductase activity	Reynafarje 1961
	Decreased fiber density per cross-sectional area	Gilbert-Kawai et al. 2014
Renal	Decrease in renal plasma and blood flow	Luks, Johnson, and Swenson 2008; Swenson and Bärtsch 2013
	Decreased glomerular filtration rate	Luks, Johnson, and Swenson 2008
	Increased filtration fraction	Luks, Johnson, and Swenson 2008
Metabolism	Rely on carbohydrates for fuel	Holden et al. 1995
	Increase glucose uptake	Woolcott, Ader, and Bergman 2015
	Lower fasting glycemia	Gerich et al. 1963
	Increased ROS production	Murray and Horscroft 2016

Data source: several.
Elaboration and analysis: authors.

In pregnant women, chronic hypoxia might diminish the rise in cardiac output, blood volume, growth, and remodeling of uterine and placental vessels. A progressive reduction in birth weight as low altitude population ascends with a mean decline in weight of 100g every 1000m of altitude gain.

Highlanders, Tibetans, Sherpas and Andeans, do not demonstrate this reduction in birth weight at altitude, in fact mean birth weights between high and low altitudes are similar. Mechanisms for pregnant and perinatal adaptation will be discussed later in the chapter.

As reviewed above, these are changes in pulmonary ventilation, increased efficiency oxygen transfer, greater total lung capacity, increased hemoglobin and RBC mass, decreased cardiac output and coronary blood flow as well as decreased venous glucose level and fasting glycemia, remodeling of uterine and placental vessels and changes in the skeletal muscle. Collectively, these are suggestive of increased efficiency oxygen distribution and utilization supporting the existence of Andean population at high altitude.

GENETIC ADAPTATION

Genetic adaptation depends on natural selection to be inherited. Natural selection is the process where the heritable traits that favor survival and reproduction become more common over time. Evolutionary forces, such as mutations, genetic drift, and gene flow also influence genetic traits (Moore 2001). Thus, when considering genetic differences between altitude regions, it is important to consider that those differences may not only be due to the effects of natural selection only but also as a result of gene flow, genetic drift or mutation. Gene flow is the transfer of genetic variation from one population to another. Genetic drift is the mechanism in which allele frequencies change over time due to chance and is inversely proportional to the size of the population. Mutation is a genetic variation that occurs randomly along the genome; single nucleotide polymorphisms (SNP) are genetic variations resulted from point mutations (Shriver et al. 2006).

Genomic studies reveal functional link between genetic regions subjected to positive selection and adaptive phenotypes of high altitude populations. Not to mention that phenotypes are the object on which selective pressures act and are seldom the product of genetic factors alone. Complex phenotypes most often arise through gene to gene and gene to environment interactions, as well as the functional interaction of the genome and epigenome. This section presents evidence supporting the possibility that genetic processes contributes to human high-altitude adaptation.

SNP genome scans and various sequencing studies have provided evidence of Andean genetic adaptation to high altitude. There is a particular interest on the genes that control or are controlled by the hypoxia-inducible factor (HIF) pathway (Julian and Moore 2019b). HIF family of transcription factors is composed by two oxygen dependent subunits: HIF-1α and HIF-2, and an oxygen independent subunit HIF-1β. HIF-1 upregulates target genes that are associated with angiogenesis, vasomotor control, erythropoiesis, apoptosis and energy metabolism (Appenzeller et al. 2006). A cell is constantly producing HIF-1/2α under normal oxygen conditions prolyl hydroxylases allows the hydroxylation of proline residues of HIF1/2α subunits, these residues are then recognized by the von Hippel–Lindau protein which marks them for ubiquitin degradation. This mechanism is regulated by the gene *EGLN1*, which acts as a molecular oxygen sensor to control hydroxylation of HIF (Bigham et al. 2010), as it encodes the oxygen sensitive prolyl hydroxylase. *EGLN1* is the only candidate gene for positive selection on both Andean and Tibetan populations, it associates with the regulation of hemoglobin on the Tibetan population, but its relation between hemoglobin and Andean population remains unknown (Heinrich et al. 2019).

In hypoxia conditions HIF-1/2α are not hydroxylated and therefore not degraded resulting in accumulation in the nucleus where it dimerises with HIF-1β to initiate gene transcription (Hochachka and Rupert 2003). This results in activation of the transcription gene that contain response elements such as genes encoding erythropoietin (*EPO*) and vascular endothelial growth factor (*VEGF*). *VEGF* is and angiogenic factor released by oxygen deprived cells. It binds flk, flt-1 and flk-4, receptor tyrosine kinases, on vascular endothelial cells resulting on proliferation of blood capillaries increasing oxygen delivery (Guillemin and Krasnow 1997).

Epigenetic regulation of HIF transcription involves silencing genes von Hippel-Lindau (*VHL*) and *EPAS*. Methylation by DNA methyltransferase 3a of *EPAS1* promoter CpG sites inhibits HIF2α gene expression in hypoxic conditions. Additionally, demethylases and histone acetyl-transferases modify the epigenetic status of histones and cytosine residues due to hypoxia, determining chromatin conformation on HIF binding sites. For this reason, epigenomic marks are expected to influence the translation of genomic sequence into physiological response

A study based on genome wide panel of 900,000 SNPs among 49 Andean and 49 Tibetan individuals for selection at high altitude identified 14 and 37 candidate regions respectively. *EDNRA, PRKAA1* and *NOS2A*, HIF pathway genes, seemed to be the best-supported candidate genes may resulted from natural selection in Andean populations. *EDNRA*, expressed in vascular smooth muscle, encodes a vasoconstrictor that is regulated through endothelin-1. *PRKAA1* encodes a heterotrimeric enzyme belonging to 5'-AMP-activated protein kinase (AMPK) gene family involved in regulation of cellular ATP. *PRKAA1* is a cellular energy sensor and protects the cells form stresses that causes ATP depletion, such as in hypoxia regulating the metabolic response to the low oxygen cellular environment (Kemp et al. 2003). *NOS2A*, synthesizes NO from arginine and oxygen. NO is a signaling molecule with various functions throughout the body, one of the functionalities related with high altitude hypoxia is the increase blood flow in the arteries regulating blood pressure, as well as smooth muscle relaxation and vasodilation (Bigham et al. 2009). Additionally, chromosome scanning in Andean populations determined that chromosomes 11, 12 and 15 had reduced variation which is an indication of directional selection. A region on chromosome 10 showed several SNPs significant different from a community of Andean highlanders compared with lowlanders. Within the region, evidence for positive selection was found on the genes *ANXA11, MAT1A, DYDC1, DYDC2, FAM213A, TSPAN14* and *SH2D4B* (Valverde et al. 2015). *FAM213A*, known as peroxiredoxin-like 2, provides protection from oxidative stress and regulates osteoclast differentiation altering bone resorption and maintaining bone mass (Xu et al. 2009). As mentioned previously, hypobaric hypoxia causes oxidative stress in the cells increasing ROS, and decreasing antioxidants (Xu et al. 2009). It suggests that antioxidants are able to protect against oxidative stress, thus, genetic factors could influence adaptive effects on the antioxidant system, as it differs between highlanders and sojourners.

Another gene identified in the analysis was *SFTPD* which encodes the lung surfactant protein D or SP-D. This works as a defense against inhaled microorganisms and acts on the extracellular remodeling or turnover of pulmonary surfactant. Besides this, *SFTPD* there are two genes associated with surfactant pulmonary proteins *SFTPA1* and SFTPA2. Mutations on these genes correlate with pulmonary fibrosis and (along with *SFTPD)* are essential for surfactant homeostasis (Choi et al. 2006). Pulmonary surfactant is essential for normal respiration, it acts as a protection against respiratory pathogens and decreases the alveoli surface tension created at the air-liquid barrier altering the surfactant surface tension during hypoxia which could be advantageous at high altitudes (Valverde et al. 2015).

Therefore, genes *VEGFB, ELTD1, BAD* and *PRDX5* were the most prominent candidates identified by haplotype homozygosity. *BAD* encodes a hypoxia responsive protein that can switch between metabolic and apoptotic functions (Danial 2008). PRDX5, a peroxisomal antioxidant enzyme that reduces hydrogen peroxide and is primarily expressed in mitochondria. *VEGFB* is a regulator of blood vessel physiology and controls endothelial uptake of fatty acids (Hagberg et al. 2010). It determined that oxygen supply can be improved by *VEGFB* which mediates angiogenesis increasing vascularization of the myocardium; *ELTD1* fundamental for cardiac development, regulates proliferation and growth of the cardiomyocytes and downregulates myocyte hypertrophy thus, seems this gene was selected to control ventricular hypertrophy. Both *VEGFB and ELTD1* are capable to modify the cardiovascular system achieving efficient blood supply controlling hypertrophy and increasing perfusion. Seems that these adaptations have co-evolved resulting in a cardiovascular system capable of counteract adverse physiological changes of living at high altitude (Eichstaedt et al. 2014).

Multifactor dimensionality reduction approach detected gene-gene interactions on *USP7, LIF, TP53* and *MDM2*. Alleles *USP7*-G and *LIF*-T are highly represented in stressful environments such us arid climate, low temperature, and high levels of UV radiation, common features of high altitudes. These SNPs have been associated with cancer, infertility, and endometriosis. Thus, these alleles *USP7*-G and *LIF*-T seem to be protective against environmental stress (Jacovas et al. 2015). MDM2, is a E3 ubiquitin protein ligase, directs p53 degradation and *MDM2* expression is in turn regulated by p53 This regulatory loop controls protein levels for MDM2 and p53 (Lozano 2016). High altitude hypoxia inhibits p53 degradation by down regulating MDM2. For this reason, literature suggest that the high expression of the alleles *MDM2-TT* genotype is an adaptation for high altitudes.

In addition, the genes *BRINP3* and *TBX5* are important for the cardiovascular system. Literature suggest an association between *BRINP3* and fibrinogen concentration. Fibrinogen concentration indicates inflammation, cardiovascular disease, arterial narrowing and blood viscosity. Low fibrinogen level is associated with an adaptive *BRINP3* allele, diminishing the effect of the allele on negative fitness. Likewise, an association between Andean allele TBX5A and a decrease on HbA1C and insulin was found; selection has favored this gene in order to restore glucose homeostasis at high altitude like increasing glycemia to normal levels (Crawford et al. 2017).

Table 2. Summary of genes that codes for genetic adaptation in Andean population

Gene	Gene name	Description*	Gene ID
EGLN1	Egl-9 family hypoxia inducible factor 1	This gene encodes a protein which catalyzes the post translational formation of 4-hydroxyproline in HIF alpha proteins	606425
EPO	Erythropoietin	This gene encodes a glycosylated cytokine of four alpha helical bundles	133170
VEGF	Vascular endothelial growth factor B	This gene encodes a member of the PDGF/VEGF family	601398
VHL	Von Hippel-Lindau tumor suppressor	This gene encodes a protein involved in ubiquitination and degradation of HIF	608537
EPAS1	Endothelial PAS domain protein 1	Encoding a transcription factor which is involved with genes regulated by oxygen	603349
EDNRA	Endothelin receptor type A	This gene encodes endothelin-1 receptor	131243
PRKAA1	Protein kinase AMP-activated catalytic subunit alpha 1	This gene encodes a protein that is a catalytic subunit of an energy sensor protein kinase	602739
NOS2A	Nitric oxide synthase 2	Encoding a nitric oxide synthase	163730
ANXA11	Annexin A11	This gene encodes a group of calcium dependent phospholipid binding proteins.	602572

Table 3. (Continued)

Gene	Gene name	Description*	Gene ID
MAT1A	Methionine adenosyltransferase 1A	This gene catalyzes a two-step reaction that result in the formation of S-adenosylmethionine and tripolyphosphate	610550
DYDC1	DPY30 domain containing 1	This gene encodes a protein that contains a DPY30 domain	615154
DYDC2	DPY30 domain containing 2	This gene encodes a protein that contains a DPY30 domain	23468
FAM213A	Family with sequence similarity 213	This gene encodes a protein which is involved in the cell redox regulation	617165
TSPAN14	Tetraspanin 14	Regulates trafficking and maturation of the transmembrane metalloprotease ADAM10	23303
SH2D4B	SH2 Domain Containing 4B	Works as an enhancer of respiratory functions	31440
SFTPD	Surfactant protein D	This gene encodes a protein which is part of the innate immune response	178635
ELTD1 (ADGRL4)	Adhesion G protein-coupled receptor L4	An endothelial orphan receptor that works as a key regulator of angiogenesis	616419
BAD	BCL2 Associated Agonist Of Cell Death	This gene encodes a protein member of the BCL-2 family, regulators of programmed cell death.	603167
PRDX5	Peroxiredoxin 5	Encoding a member of the peroxiredoxin family of antioxidant enzymes	606583
USP7	Ubiquitin Specific Peptidase 7	This gene encodes a protein that belongs to the peptidase C19 family	602519
LIF	LIF Interleukin 6 Family Cytokine	This gene encodes a protein which is a pleiotropic cytokine.	159540
TP53	Tumor Protein P53	Encoding a tumor suppressor protein that contains transcriptional activation, oligomerization domains and DNA binding.	191170
MDM2	MDM2 Proto-Oncogene	This gene encodes a E3 ubiquitin ligase	164785
BRINP3	BMP/Retinoic Acid Inducible Neural Specific 3	This gene regulates the cell cycle transition	618390
TBX5	T-Box 5	This gene is a member of the T-box phylogenetically conserved genes family.	601620
ACE	Angiotensin I Converting Enzyme	This gene encodes a catalytic enzyme involved in the conversion of angiotensin I into angiotensin II	106180

Data source: *Definitions accessed from NCBI database.
Elaboration and analysis: authors.

Whole genome sequencing (WGS) identified angiotensin converting enzyme (ACE) as implicated in high-altitude adaptation. ACE is a central component of the renin-angiotensin-aldosterone (RAS) system involved in the regulation of cardiovascular homeostasis. Two different alleles have been determined; insertion (I) allele correlates with lower ACE protein function, whereas deletion (D) allele with enhanced ACE activity of which the predominant on high altitude natives is the I allele. D allele has been related with high altitude pulmonary edema (Bhagi et al. 2015). Thus, I allele might be playing an advantageous role on adaptation to high altitude (Tomar, Malhotra, and Sarkar 2015).

Pregnancy and Perinatal Adaptation

High altitude environment challenges human life due to temperature changes but especially due to lower partial pressure of oxygen in the atmosphere. In fact, this high altitude exacerbates the extreme surrounding that an intrauterine environment possess (Shao 2019; Gassmann et al. 2016). High altitude pregnancies are a burden for both mother and fetus as the risk of pregnancy complications and neonatal morbidity increases. Intrauterine growth restriction (IUGR), aberrant organ development, neurobehavioral disorders in neonates, impaired fetal growth, increased risk of preeclampsia are some of the complications that have been shown to occur (Shao 2019).

During pregnancy, the pregnant women undergoes physiological and anatomical changes in order to nurture and accommodate the fetus. One of the physiological challenges for fetal development is to maintain an adequate supply of oxygenated blood to the uteroplacental circulation (Julian 2011). As pregnant women and their unborn children respond differently to high altitude hypoxia, due to fetal arterial oxygen tensions in the utero are low by adult standards seen even under normal conditions (Shao 2019). Thus, a pregnant woman exposed briefly, intermittently, or permanently to high altitude results on increased risk of adverse outcomes when it compares to pregnancies observed at sea level (Gonzales 2012).

Interestingly, congenital defects (CD) rates are higher at high altitudes. The more frequent defects occur in locomotion organs (29%), the facial region (16%) and the cardiovascular system (12%) (Gonzales 2012). Besides, it seems that there is an association between high altitude pregnancy and increased frequency of congenital heart disease (CHD) (García et al. 2016). CHD, is a birth defect that includes heart structure abnormalities, with significant risk of mortality (Hasan 2016). Critical congenital heart disease (CCHD) occurs every 40 newborns per 10,000 live newborns (LNB), where 13-55% of newborns were discharge undiagnosed. Pulse oximetry is a non-invasive low-cost test that aids the diagnose CCHD (Kim et al. 2018) so that newborns can benefit from early diagnosis and treatment (Paranka et al. 2018). Antenatal ultrasound and newborn physical examination are used as screening strategies for the diagnose of CCHD however, both have low detection rates. Thereby, infants are discharged undiagnosed. Pulse oximetry allows to detect hypoxemia in the absence of clinical cyanosis, discoloration of the skin (Tin and Lal 2015). It is now recommended screening tool for CCHD with a cutoff SpO2 of 95% (Kim et al. 2018). However, mean pulse oximetry values at moderate and high altitude locations are lower than the cutoffs for newborn screening (Kim et al. 2018; González-Andrade et al. 2018b). For this reason, utilizing this screening method at moderate to high altitudes will result in false positive results. A study from moderate altitude in Aurora, USA (at 1694 masl) showed high failure rates of pulse oximetry screening compared to those at sea level, even with a cut-off value of 90%(Kim et al. 2018). Until now, CHD occurrence at high altitude worldwide remains lacking.(Li et al. 2019).

Thus, two approaches have been suggested for screening infants at altitude and to limit the false positive rate. First, providing oxygen to correct for the impact lower oxygen availability in the alveoli, or second, adjusting and testing the pulse oximetry parameters based the population being evaluated. Even though, both solutions look promising, further research needs to be done.

During pregnancy, maternal and fetal physiological compensations for decreased oxygen availability results in a successful pregnancy outcome (Julian 2011). The physiology of healthy women living at high altitude is able to counteract the arterial hypoxia and aid hemodynamic adaptations to increase utero-placental blood flow by increasing maternal ventilation rate and oxygen blood saturation level. Therefore, the developing fetus is able to cope with the oxygen reduced supply occurring in the utero. (Gassmann et al. 2016). In fact, at high altitude pregnant Andean women have increased levels of arterial oxygen and higher utero-placental blood flow compared to Europeans (Julian 2011). Likewise, vasodilation occurs and microvascular density is higher on neonates born to mothers living at high altitude than in neonates born at sea level.

Moreover, perinatal Doppler and ultrasound studies at 3,600masl in Andean fetuses determined that reduced umbilical blood flow is compensated by an increase on neonatal hemoglobin concentration and greater fetuses oxygen extraction capability (Postigo et al. 2009). Thus, values for fetal oxygen delivery and consumption at high altitude are not different to the ones at low altitude, suggesting that the fetus copes with the extreme environment in utero. Indeed, most Andean fetuses develop properly and are delivered at term.

On the other hand, the fetus physiology allows adaptation for intrauterine environment being significantly different from the neonate. Transition to extrauterine life involves various complex processes to ensure survival, characterized by changes in circulatory pathways, initiation of ventilation and oxygenation via the lungs instead of the placenta, and various metabolism alterations (Morton and Brodsky 2016). Prior birth, the placenta is a low resistance area that ensures low pressure deoxygenated blood returns for exchange, while the lungs are on an area of high resistance thus, pulmonary flow is diverted. The placenta receives 40% of fetal cardiac output whereas fetal lungs receive approximately 10% of cardiac output (Swanson and Sinkin 2015). Since oxygenated maternal blood mixes with poor oxygenated blood in the placental space, the blood oxygen concentration provided to the fetus is lower than the maternal uterine arterial blood, inducing the fetus to live in a hypoxic environment. Not to mention that fetal lungs do not contribute to intrauterine oxygenation, thus, intrauterine shunts are designed to lead blood away from the fetal lungs (Morton and Brodsky 2016). These fetal shunts not only to divert blood away from fetal lungs but also from less critical organs like gut and kidneys to direct it to organs that are critical for survival such as the heart brain and adrenal glands (Graves and Haley 2013).

Additionally, the placenta provides the fetus with oxygen and nutrients via the umbilical vein. The umbilical vein divides at the liver with some blood to perfuse the hepatic circulation and the remainder enters the ductus venosus. Most of the blood from the ductus venosus is directed to the left atrium, the inferior and superior vena cava blood enters the right atrium. Right ventricular output is directed into the descending aorta across the patent ductus arteriosus (PDA). Left ventricular output provides blood flow to the preductal vessels supplying the coronary arteries, the brain and upper body. Intrauterine pulmonary blood flow is initially limited because of the high pulmonary vascular resistance and the right-to-left shunting across the patent foramen ovale and PDA (Morton and Brodsky 2016).

Blood reaching the intrauterine pulmonary circulation has an oxygenation saturation of approximately 55% due to favored shunting of deoxygenated blood into the right ventricle. Hypoxia decreases fetal pulmonary blood flow, that in turn represses nitric oxide and prostaglandin I2 production. Resulting, in an elevated pulmonary vascular resistance at baseline. Any additional fetal hypoxemia increases pulmonary vascular resistance activating HIF-1 and triggering vascular remodeling. HIF-1 stimulates the fetal kidneys to produce EPO, increasing RBC production, improving oxygenation of the fetus. This enhanced EPO leads to increase hematocrit and hemoglobin concentration in the cord blood. Additionally, fetal hemoglobin has high oxygen affinity, shifting left the oxyhemoglobin curve to augment oxygen uptake at the lower oxygenated placental vascular bed (Morton and Brodsky 2016). In fact, the ratio of fetal hemoglobin in the cord blood is elevated at high altitude compared to sea level populations.

From the cardiovascular point of view, transition to extrauterine environment involves an increment on the systemic vascular resistance and pulmonary blood flow, decreased pulmonary vascular resistance, closure of right to left shunts, fetal lung resorption and expansion. Further changes occur after delivery due to the removal of the resistance placenta as the source of fetal gas exchange and nutrition. Increasing cardiac output and transition to an adult-type of circulation (Hillman, Kallapur, and Jobe 2012).

A newborn with CHD is not always diagnosed before birth, because at some locations prenatal diagnosis is not routinely offered, thereby birth is the only moment when a heart anomaly could be diagnosed depending on the presented symptoms. The first few breaths of a healthy baby inflate the lungs, lowering the circulatory system resistance thus, increasing pulmonary blood flow (Morton and Brodsky 2016). Then, the umbilical cord is cut blocking the placental low-pressure, increasing the systemic vascular resistance in the newborn. Left-sided atrial pressure increases rapidly due to a severe rise in left atrial return from the pulmonary veins, closing the septal layers of the foramen ovale. Then, the ductus arteriosus will gradually close. Oxygenation of the ductus arteriosus increments calcium channel activity leading to a functional closure. Smooth muscle cells of the ductus arteriosus inhibit potassium channel activity as a response to increased oxygen enhancing ductal constriction. The timing of umbilical cord clamping seems to be essential. Delays in cord clamping until the onset of ventilation prevents this decrease in cardiac output. In most babies' gas exchange is stabilized by 2 minutes after vaginal delivery utilizing the improvement in heart rate as a clinical indicator proper ventilation (Webb, Perkins, and Ketty 2016). Besides, by 24 hours of age pulmonary arterial pressure reaches half the systemic arterial pressure, reaching adult levels in two weeks (Gao and Raj 2009). After, this transition the full return of deoxygenated blood into the right heart is directed to the lungs for oxygenation, followed by the full return of oxygenated blood from the lungs directed to the body and tissues.

In contrast, this cardiopulmonary transition differs at high altitude location compared to sea level because of the fundamental role that oxygen plays in the changes from fetus to neonate. For example, impaired cardiopulmonary transition after birth is more frequently at high altitude characterized by lower and highly variable arterial oxygen saturation compared to sea level (Niermeyer 2003). Under hypoxia, arterial oxygen saturations are lower, thus, maturation of respiratory control reflexes, breathing patterns and regression of the pulmonary vasculature advance slowly. As seen geographical location plays a significant role in congenital heart disease as high altitude hypoxia changes the heart chamber dynamic pressure altering the hemodynamic adaptation of neonatal circulation (Hasan 2016). Oxygen is essential in and birth into a high altitude hypoxic environment has connotations that may extend throughout life

Even though, inspired oxygen tension is important for infant's arterial oxygen saturation, it also depends on various physiological variables, such as respiratory rate, oxyhemoglobin binding, and the pulmonary vascular bed. Infants within the first hours of birth at sea level achieve SaO2 between 96% and 98%. Whereas at 2850masl at Quito, Ecuador, values of preductal oxygen saturation in healthy neonates were from 89.74% to 95.8%; and postductal saturation was from 90.93% to 96.5% (González-Andrade et al. 2018). At extreme high altitude in Peru (4540 masl), arterial oxygen saturations range from 57% to 75%, in infants from 30 min to 72 hours of age. Suggesting an indirect relationship, where that oxygen saturation decreases as altitude increases (González-Andrade et al. 2018; Paranka et al. 2018). These populations differences in arterial oxygen saturation suggests a role for genetic adaptation.

PATHOLOGICAL MECHANISMS OF CONGENITAL HEART DISEASE

High altitude is a risk factor for CHD (Chun et al. 2018). The embryonic development of the human heart requires multiple complex and time-dependent processes, that need to occur in a proper order to prevent structural and functional abnormalities such as CHD. Heart development depends on cellular proliferation, differentiation, migration, and morphogenesis of cardiac structures. Cardiac progenitor cells differentiate into cell subtypes such as fibroblasts, cardiomyocytes, valvular interstitial cells, conduction system, pericardium and endocardium, others (Kloesel, DiNardo, and Body 2016).

In humans, at 15-16 days of gestation heart development begins and occurs in five steps. First, precardiac cells migrates from the primitive streak and at the myocardial plate assembles the paired cardiac crescents. Second, formation of the primitive heart tube by the cardiac crescents. Third, cardiac looping ensures adequate alignment of the future cardiac chambers. Fourth, septation and formation of the heart chambers. Fifth, the development of coronary vasculature and conduction system (Huang, Liu, and Lv 2010).

Cells involved in the development of the heart are derived from three precursor populations, cardiac neural crest cells, cardiogenic-mesoderm cells, and proepicardial cells.

The heart tube is formed through fusion in the midline following lateral folding of the embryonic disk from the first heart field cells. Then, a rearrangement of the endocardial tube position is essential for four heart chambers formation as well as the inflow and outflow connections to the vasculature. The cardiogenic genes NKX2.5, SRF, GATA4, TBX5, and

HAND2, constitute the main network of cardiac morphogenesis regulators, which controls heart looping, side symmetry, and chambers formation (Dunwoodie 2007). Cardiac looping is driven by the endocardial tube leads to the formation of the atria and right ventricle parts and the early left ventricle. In the process of left-right body axis determination is crucial to avoid disruptions to prevent laterality disorders, ranging from abnormal positioning to absence of internal organs. The final step is the septation of the primitive ventricles and outflow tract into systemic and pulmonary trunks.

The development of the efferent pathway involves neural crest cells, the endocardium and the myocardium. simultaneous and intricate process occur, such as epithelia-mesenchymal transition of the endocardium to form the endocardial cushions, neural crest cells colonization of the extracellular matrix, and finally the rotation of the myocardium to align vessels with their respective ventricle wedging (Bajolle, Zaffran, and Bonnet 2009). At day 21, the primitive heart begins to beat and blood pumping starts by day 24-25,while the heart mature by day 50. Where Chemotaxis, chemical signals, from surrounding or distant cells and mechanotaxis, mechanical signals, from neighbor cells play an important role to determine cell fate (Kloesel, DiNardo, and Body 2016). Additionally, hemodynamic forces have been shown to play a valuable function in cardiac development. Impaired forces or defects on the regulation of the genes involved in growth and differentiation, defects may arise. The increase of environmental oxygen levels in neonates seems to be effective in stimulating spontaneous closure of ductus arteriosus thus, declining the incidence of patent ductus arteriosus and early mortality from unrestrictive ventricular septal defect (Zheng et al. 2017).

The most common CHD is the bicuspid aortic valve affecting 1-2% of the population (Mordi and Tzemos 2012; Freeze et al. 2016; Huang, Liu, and Lv 2010). After bicuspid aortic valve, ductus arteriosus patency, septal defects, and great arteries anomalies are the most frequent CHD, with increased incidence at high altitude. Phenotypes of CHD can vary from a small atrial-septal defect (ASD) and a ventricular-septal defect (VSD), that may go undetected throughout life, to large ASD and VSD which are symptomatic. Within clinically anomalies ranges from complex defects like transposition of the great vessels, single ventricle anomaly, hypoplastic left heart syndrome, and complex variants of heterotaxy to a more simple persistence of fetal circulation such as patent ductus arteriosus.

According to the pathogenetic classification of CHD, there are six causative mechanisms: First, ecto-mesenchymal tissue migration abnormalities. Second, intracardiac blood flow defects. Third, cell death abnormalities. Fourth, extracellular matrix defects. Fifth, targeted growth abnormalities. Lastly, situs and looping defects (Huang, Liu, and Lv 2010). In the other hand, prevalence of CHD in newborns at high altitude is about 20 times higher than at low altitude, consisting mostly of simple forms with left to right shunt, with rare complex CHD. By 12 to18 months of age, the prevalence of CHD is still about 10 times higher than that at low altitude (Li et al. 2019). Decreased oxygen tension at high altitude has been postulated as critical in the observed increase in patency of ductus arteriosus at birth, and hypoxia has been implicated as an extrinsic factor for defective embryogenesis in CHD. Interventricular defects and atrial septal defects have also been associated with altitude. Previous studies postulated a reasonable pathophysiologic mechanism by which persistently high pulmonary pressures at high altitude after birth could inhibit patent foramen ovale closure and predispose to atrial defects (García et al. 2016).

High prevalence of PDA at high altitudes determined that oxygen tension is a major factor of patency, and spontaneous closure of the ductus arteriosus. At high altitude, low oxygen tension may inhibit the spontaneous closure, allowing the ductus arteriosus to remain patent. Children with PDA-dependent complex heart disease could survive at high altitudes due to the persistent patency of a large ductus (Zheng et al. 2017). Altitude not only had an effect on PDA but also on the prevalence of ASD. The reason for children high prevalence of ASD at high altitude remains unknown. However, one of the theories suggest that the inhibited early closure of the foramen ovale is due to the persistence of high pulmonary vascular resistance and right heart pressure. Subsequent formation of an atrial septal defect due to growth resulting on stretching of the fossa ovalis and incompetence of the flap (Zheng et al. 2017).

In low altitude regions, PDA almost always closes by three to four days after birth, while 85 - 90% of muscular VSD and ASD close spontaneously by 1 year of age. At high altitude in postnatal newborns three to five days the prevalence of PDA was more than twice in comparison to those at sea level. Where 83.7% closing by three months. At twelve to eighteen months, 11.8% PDA, 33.7% ASD, and 23.1% VSD remained open (Li et al. 2019). Unfortunately, at high altitude few CHD patients are offered surgical treatment or interventional repair at time. An early detection of CHD is critical to improve survival.

Atrial Septal Defect

Atrial septal defects (ASDs) are a common form of CHD representing 10% of all CHD. This defect usually is sporadic but occasionally can be familial. The atrial septum, heterogeneous structure, separates 2 atrial chambers. Impairments of any of these structures may lead to ASDs resulting in a communication between the left and right atria, clinically known as a shunt (Gruber and Epstein 2004). ASD divides into patent foramen ovale, ostium secundum defect ost,ium primum defect, sinus venosus defect, common atrium and coronary sinus defect. If there is a shunt in early postnatal life, is normally diagnosed after the extra-uterine circulation transition because of the decrease in the pulmonary vascular resistance (PVR) and the increase in systemic vascular resistance (SVR) causing the manifestation of left to right shunts in the form of congestive heart failure (CHF) (Chowdhury 2009).

In highlanders, the time at which PVR lowers in highlanders is usually longer than in lowlanders thus, ASD has been found to be of prevalence at high altitudes (Hasan 2016). A persistent left to-right shunt of blood results in growth of the right ventricle and atrium, as well as atrial arrhythmias, ventricular impairment, and pulmonary over-circulation deriving irreversible pulmonary vascular obstructive disease. The life expectancy for patients with significant big shunts is 45 years. Thus, by the age of 3-4 years children with ASDs should have them closed.

There has been identified some the genetic causes of some forms of ASD. For example, Holt-Oram syndrome patients usually have ASDs associated with limb deformities. Due to mutations in the gene *TBX5*, a T-box transcription factor gene whereas in patients with isolated ASDs it was found mutations in *GATA4*. Both genes can physically interact suggesting regulation within a transcriptional complex may contribute to atrial septal formation. Literature also determined that *TBX, GATA4*, and *NKX2-5* act at several stages of cardiac development (Gruber and Epstein 2004).

Besides, patent foramen ovale (PFO) is a small communication between left and right atria. Even though it is considered benign at sea level, evidence suggest that PFO is frequently associated with ischemic stroke, migraines, decompression sickness and peripheral embolism. Especially, in high altitude residents due to the higher pulmonary and heart pressure, a PFO may have complications. Patients with a PFO are more susceptible to reversal of flow across. In fact, literature determines that a PFO in highlanders correlates with right ventricular growth and dysfunction and an exaggerated increase in PAP at mild exercises.(Li et al. 2019).

Ventricular Septal Defect

Ventricular septal defects (VSDs) are another form of CHD. VSDs are the most common non valvular CHD affecting to 0.5% of population. Most are minimal and close spontaneously without treatment but VSD are a frequent factor of more complex lesions. VSD was the most frequent feature observed CHD at low and intermediate altitudes (García et al. 2016). Besides, an unrestricted VSD creates susceptibility for pulmonary hypertension at high altitude compared with sea level.

VSDs are usually classified by their location and may occur in the ventricular septum. VSDs are classified into membranous ventricular septal defect, inlet ventricular septal defect, muscular ventricular septal defect and infundibular VSD (Kloesel, DiNardo, and Body 2016). Most of the cases are non-symptomatic, thus diagnosis of VSD is initially suspected based on the physical examination alone (Gruber and Epstein 2004).

There is a left to right shunt across the ventricular level occurring at systole (high pressure) where blood from left ventricle (LV) to be eject in systole to the pulmonary circulation causing a volume overload to the left atrium and the LV. In VSD the left to right shunt is more significant driving the progression towards pulmonary vascular disease sooner. The right ventricular (RV) pressure is determined by the size of the VSD (Chowdhury 2009). There an increased susceptibility to develop pulmonary hypertension in children with VSD at high altitude compared to sea level (Zheng et al. 2017).

There are various possible mechanisms leading to anomalies due to the heterogeneous composition of the ventricular septum. The compex region of the ventricular septum is the anterior and the superior where, the muscular ventricular crest joins the atrioventricular cushions and the cono-truncal cushions. Also, there are important transitory structures for cardiac septation.

Patent Ductus Arteriosus

The fetal vascular connection between the main pulmonary artery and the aorta is known as the ductus arteriosus (DA). It works as a right-to-left shunt allowing placental oxygenated blood to bypass the non-ventilated lungs and reach the systemic circulation (Iwashima et al. 2018). After birth the ductal closure occurs in two steps. First, functional closure, the significant increase in oxygen tension and decrease prostaglandin (PGE2) levels from the placenta constrain ductal smooth muscle voltage-dependent potassium channels, and results in an influx of calcium and thus ductal constriction. Likewise, the postpartum elevation in arterial oxygen tension enhances a ductal constrictor mechanism. Second, anatomical closure involves tissue remodeling resulting in permanent structural closure.

Contraction of medial smooth muscle fibers in the ductus results in wall thickening, shortening of the ductus arteriosus and lumen obliteration. A complete functional closure occurs within 24 -48 hours after birth in term neonates and the DA closes in 3 days. The subsequent 2-3 weeks results in a permanent seal by the formation of fibrosis through endothelium unfolding along with subintimal disruption and proliferation. This resulting fibrous band persists as the ligamentum arteriosum. If the DA fails to completely close after birth PDA occurs. A high prevalence is found in preterm low birth weight infants and most patients are non-symptomatic when the duct is small (Forsey, Elmasry, and Martin 2009).

There is a left to right shunt during diastole and systole from the aorta to the pulmonary artery. Pulmonary artery pressures are lower in systole and diastole compared to the aorta resulting in a continuous shunt (Chowdhury 2009). Adult PDA occurs sporadically one in 2000 individuals, but associations related with condition identified such as chromosomal abnormalities, which found in 8-11% of cases of PDA. It is also associated with chromosomal aberrations, birth at high altitude (Gonzales 2012), asphyxia at birth and congenital rubella (Forsey, Elmasry, and Martin 2009). PDA is a common defect found at high altitude. The type of PDA at highland is different than at lowland, presenting with a larger ductal diameter.

Atrioventricular Canal

Atrioventricular canal (AVC), known as endocardial cushion defect, affects over 1 in 2800 LNB, being 7,4% of all CHDs (Digilio et al. 2019). The most common variations comprise a combination of defects in the atrial septum primum, ventricular septum inlet portion, and a common atrioventricular canal (CAVC). CAVC lesions can be partial, transitional or complete. In case it is undiagnosed during the neonatal period, these infants usually present CHF due to a large left-to-right shunt, that increases as the pulmonary vascular resistance decreases (Gruber and Epstein 2004).

A primary intracardiac mechanism consisting in the anomal development of endocardial cushions related to defects of extracellular matrix was considered the cause of an AVC with absent or incomplete fusion of atrioventricular cushions ventrally and dorsally. However, recent studies have determined that disturbance of extracardiac tissue, extracardial mesenchymal cells known as dorsal mesocardial protrusion (DMP), is a major determinant of AVC (Digilio et al. 2019). These cells arise from the posterior segment of the secondary heart field in the splanchnic mesoderm and migrate to the atrial surface of the primitive AVC, in order to close the primary atrial foramen and thus form the AV junction. Surgical repair can be performed at three to six months.

Cardiac Outflow Tract Anomalies

Cardiac outflow tract anomalies represent a panel of heart developmental disorders with common etiologic features. Cardiac neural crest cells are crucial for shaping the outflow tract by controlling the remodeling process. Impairment of neural crest cell induction, specification, endothelial to mesenchymal transition, cell-cell interaction, migration, and condensation to form the outflow tract explain the major factor in the origin of anomaly conditions, such as tetralogy of Fallot, persistent truncus arteriosus (PTA), transposition of the great arteries, and double-outlet right ventricle (Kloesel, DiNardo, and Body 2016).

Persistent Truncus Arteriosus

Persistent truncus arteriosus (PTA), is a defect in the septum formation that divides the truncus arteriosus into aorta and pulmonary artery, resulting on one combined blood outflow tract ejected by each ventricle. The truncal valve is structurally abnormal and a VSD is present in almost all cases. PTA is an uncommon form of CHD, affecting one in 10,000 live neonates. Right aortic arch, arch hypoplasia, aortic coarctation, and interruption are common extracardiac and cardiac abnormalities. For the first week of live infants with PTA show symptoms of CHF and may be cyanotic.

At high altitude there is a slower rate of decrease in PVR so that neonates at higher altitudes are able to maintain high pulmonary vein resistance for a longer period of time. Thereby, symptoms may appear later than expected (Chowdhury 2009). A microdeletion of chromosome 22 has been recorded on one third of patients with PTA. This deletion is associated with DiGeorge syndrome, which comprises parathyroid, thymus and cardiovascular defects and craniofacial abnormalities.

Besides, the gene *TBX1* is involved cardiac development on chromosome 22, surrounding genes may regulate *TBX1* function or cause PTA independently. Neural crest cells, multipotent cell population specified in the dorsal neural tube, function in truncal septation and aids in the developing outflow tract of the heart. These cells differentiate into the smooth muscle of the aortic arch and ductus arteriosus.

Transposition of Great Arteries

Transposition of great arteries (TGA) is a frequent cyanotic lesion that appears during the first week of life, it affect one in 3,100 live newborns. In TGA, the pulmonary artery arises from the left ventricle and the aorta from the right ventricle resulting in a separate parallel, pulmonary and systemic circulations. Thus, a communication between the left and right sides via a PDA, PFO, ASD or VSD is essential for survival. Literature suggest a role for neural crest in the pathogenesis of TGA, but it is poorly understood

Coronary artery abnormal positioning is a frequent deffect occurring in a third of patients whereas VSD occurs on 25% of the patients, ASDs on 10%, aortic arch abnormalities on 5%, and tricuspid valve abnormalities on 4% (Gruber and Epstein 2004).

Dextro-transposition of the great arteries (D-TGA), is the relationship of the ventricles to the atria after cardiac looping to the right. It presents concordant atrioventricular and discordant ventriculo-arterial connections. On the contrary, corrected transposition has to be consider strictly separated from D-transposition due to its different pathophysiology and pathogenesis.

Double Outlet Right Ventricle

Double-outlet right ventricle (DORV) is an uncommon group of defects that is characterized by both great vessels, aorta and pulmonary artery, arising from the right ventricle (Gruber and Epstein 2004). During outflow tract development, poor alignment defects drives the development of a DORV. The aortic-pulmonary septum develops normally and separates the great vessels, but incorrect alignment of the aorta over the right ventricle results in a position that both great vessels arise from the right ventricle.

Children with DORV is presented in a wide range of ways depending on the relationship of the great vessels to the VSD, if outflow obstruction is present, and the size of the left ventricle. DORV is commonly associated with a VSD and pulmonary stenosis due to a right-to-left shunt after birth (Kloesel, DiNardo, and Body 2016).

Tetralogy of Fallot

Tetralogy of Fallot (TOF) is a form of cyanotic CHD during infancy. During fetal development, anterior and cephalad displacement of the infundibular septum describe VSD and right ventricular outflow tract obstruction (RVOTO) in TOF. (Karl and Stocker 2016). The four distinguishing elements are VSD, overriding of the aorta, RV hypertrophy, and RV outflow obstruction. TOF occurs sporadically and the genetic etiology is remains unknwon. The main cause of TOF is poorly understood, however, there are theories associating it with 22q11.2 deletion syndrome as well as rare copy number variations of *TBX1, SNX8, PLXNA2, NOTCH1,* and *JAG1*.

Heterotaxy

Disorders involving a defective left-right axis determination that results in atypical positioning of internal organs. Impairment of positional axis formation occurs at the third week of embryonic develpment. Defect in the left-right axis impacts the unique arrangement of thoracic and visceral organs in organism. Right isomerism includes absence of a spleen (asplenia), bilateral trilobed lungs, and complex cardiovascular abnormalities requiring uni-ventricular repair. Left isomerism is characterized by the presence of multiple spleens, called polysplenia; bilateral bilobed lungs, and less complex cardiovascular abnormalities that can be addressed with bi-ventricular repair (Shiraishi and Ichikawa 2012). Additionally, patients with heterotaxy are susceptible to arrhythmias. Tachycardias are common patients with left isomerism, atrial tachycardia, atrial flutter junctional tachycardia, ventricular tachycardia, supraventricular tachycardia. While, patients with right isomerism showed frequent conduction blocks, complete AV block, intra-ventricular conduction delay, sick sinus syndrome.

Anomalies of the Aortic Arch

Congenital aortic arch defects with a large range of variations and anomalies that emanate from disordered branchial arches. It includes anomalies such as coarctation of aorta, vascular rings and interrupted aortic arch. Either abnormal persistence or involution of vascular segments result on these aberrations (Priya et al. 2018) Most of the defects related to the disruption of aortic depends on the PDA. The fact that DA remains open for a longer period of time at high altitude, the diagnosis could be delayed.

The development of the normal aorta and its branches starts with six pairs of pharyngeal arches that connects the two primitive ventral and dorsal aortas. This development begins at the second week of gestation until the seventh week. The two dorsal aortas fuse and form a single vessel, while the six pairs of aortic arches appear and regress at different times. First the aortic arches I and II form disappear, then aortic arch III and part of the ventral and dorsal aortic arches form the common carotid arteries. Aortic arch IV becomes the aortic arch while aortic arch V never fully develops. Finally, the distal part of the right aortic arch VI disappears, the left proportion persist as DA, the proximal portion forms the right pulmonary artery (RPA) while the proximal portion of the left aortic arch VI forms the left pulmonary artery (LPA). Migration of the intersegmental arteries form the subclavian arteries. (S. Li et al. 2019).

Aortic Coarctation

Aortic coarctation is a CHD whereby the aorta is narrow. The location of this constriction is limited to the entire length. However, it is frequently found at the origin of the left subclavian artery and the DA. It occurs three cases per 10,000 live newborns. (Cangussú, Lopes, and Barbosa 2019). Aortic coarctation is divide into two distinct groups: critical aortic coarctation and asymptomatic aortic coarctation. In the critical coarctation, is characterized by severe symptoms in the first two months of life and if left untreated leads to death. The asymptomatic coarctation is characterized by the late onset of hypertension on upper limbs. During embryogenic development, coarctation is not well understood. But, theories suggest that there a disorder migration of DA smooth muscle cells to the wall of the aorta artery while others suggest a change of blood flow in the fetal circulation, that decrease the amount of blood in the left ventricle to the aorta.

Interrupted Aortic Arch

Interrupted aortic arch (IAA) is a congenital vascular defect with discontinuity between the ascending aorta (AAO) and descending aorta (DAO). It represents only 1% of all CHD. IAA is similar to aortic coarctation, but the underlaying mechanisms are different. This defect is commonly associated with posterior incorrect alignment of the infundibular septum with the muscular septum. There are three anatomic subtypes of interrupted aortic arch which are based on the location of the interruption. Type A distal to the left subclavian artery. Type B is between a subclavian artery and a carotid artery. Type C between the two carotid arteries.

Hypoplastic Left Heart Syndrome

Hypoplastic left heart syndrome (HLHS) is a group of anatomic abnormalities with a small or absent left ventricle with aortic valves and hypoplastic ascending aorta and hypoplastic or atretic mitral. Two shunts must be present for the newborn to survive. One shunt at the atrial level allows mixing of pulmonary venous blood with blood in the right atrium, and the second shunt, an intact DA, provides flow and retrograde flow to the systemic circulation and coronary arteries, respectively.

For survival, a pathway of palliation is possible through a series operations resulting in a Fontan circulation (Roeleveld et al. 2018). After birth, palliation can be undertaken by staged operations: In the first week of life Norwood, at four to six month of life a superior cavopulmonary connection, and at 2 to 4 yoears of life a total cavopulmonary connection.

Success and progression to these surgeries are challenging at high altitude due to the increase of PVR. There is risk of circulatory failure their entire life, and selected patients may undergo heart transplantation. Patients with single ventricle and postoperative staged surgeries do not tolerate high altitude due to hypoxia (Hasan 2016).

Pulmonary Atresia with VSD

Pulmonary atresia with ventricular septal defect (PA/VSD) is a rare disease in which the ventricles size are normal but there is usually a severe hypoplastic infundibulum with complete atresia of the pulmonary valve. It seems that genetic pathways involved in DiGeorge syndrome and the development of cardiac outflow tract are similar to pathways disrupted in PA/VSD.

Etiological Mechanisms of Congenital Heart Diseases

Despite research undertaken to understand of cardiac development and the identification of many genes related to cardiac development, the fundamental etiology for the majority of cases of CHD remains unknown. Literature describe several risk factors such as, folic acid insufficiency, increased nuchal translucency in first trimester, assisted reproductive technology, maternal diabetes or obesity, maternal hypertension, maternal anti-hypertensive medication, among others. Even though more than 50% of cases etiology are still unknown, genetic causes produce approximately 45% of both isolated and syndromic CHD. Ten percent of severe CHD are cause by De novo point mutations, and familial CHD (least 3 generations) have 30% of pathogenic variants (Zaidi 2017). Additionally, they have associated comorbidities, such as extracardiac anomalies in 25% of cases and developmental disability affects 10% of all CHD, 50% in severe cases.

The low heritability patterns suggest that environmental factors, such as altitude, rather than genetic factors, play am essential role in the incidence of CHD (Chun et al. 2018). Non-genetic causes for impairment of normal heart development includes viral infections, maternal exposure to alcohol, drugs, environmental teratogens, metabolic disturbances (Kloesel, DiNardo, and Body 2016), rubella, measles, exposure to chemicals maternal systemic lupus erythematosus (Huang, Liu, and Lv 2010).

Epidemiologic studies of CHD suggest an increment recurrence risk for CHD in sequential pregnancies as it may support genetic predisposition. Nevertheless, tracing the disease to its precise etiology is difficult. Not to mention that anomalies or defects are thought to be because an priori genetic predisposition which will in turn enhance the effect of any exposure to a teratogen (Sandridge et al. 2011) However, an association between specific mutations of a gene controlling cardiac development, with a heart malformation does not occur most of the time.

In fact, less than 20% of CHD diseases can be explained by chromosomal defects or single-gene disorders. Despite the fact that many genetic and epigenetics mechanisms are not yet understood. Penetrance of disease gene mutations is known, and these studies provided 3notable insights First, human CHD disease mutations impact a heterogeneous panel of molecules involved in cardiac development, second, CHD mutations seems often alter gene-protein dosage, and third, identical pathogenic CHD mutations results on distinct defects.

CHD occurs during embryogenesis acquiring de novo somatic gene mutation or by inheritance of a gene mutation from a parent. Abnormal chromosome structures single nucleotide polymorphisms, gene mutations, abnormal RNA, and epigenetics are known to be the origin of CHD. The marked heterogeneity found in various CHD groups increase the complexity, however, it has allowed the analysis and association of phenotype- genotype relationships (Bajolle, Zaffran, and Bonnet 2009).

On the other hand, epigenetics describes changes that occur in the transcriptional stage of cells which are not directly caused by alterations in the DNA itself. Epigenetics includes the DNA and chromatin modifications involved in regulation of various genomic functions. Certainly, the genotype the majority of cells in a given organism is the same, except gametes and immune system cells, cellular functionality differ thoroughly. This can be controlled to some extent by epigenetic regulation.

CHD have heterogeneous pathophysiologic mechanisms, that as technology in molecular biology and genetics develops, greater insight and knowledge can be gained (Kloesel, DiNardo, and Body 2016). Impaired embryonic cardiac development mechanism may produce anatomically and structurally different cardiac phenotypes. Thus, genetic counselling for CHD is based on the process and mechanism of a given heart defect rather than its anatomy (Bajolle, Zaffran, and Bonnet 2009).

The role of high altitude as an environmental determinant of CHD has been proposed for the past 60 years in different ways, being a feature of embryonic tissue hypoxia or an important risk factor at the time of delivery at high altitude. However, in the case of PDA or ASD, its suggested that could be related to a persistence of pulmonary hypertension rather than a congenital defect. Even though some cases of PDA are predominantly associated with genetics, the increased prevalence at high altitudes suggest a leading role for such environmental mechanisms that are mediated by low atmospheric pressure (García et al. 2016).

THE CASE OF ECUADOR: LIVING ABOVE 2500 MASL

Ecuador is located in South America, and reached 17 million inhabitants in 2019. It is a unique country mainly for three reasons; first, it is demographically multi-ethnic and multi-cultural with three main ethnic groups, and 13 native nationalities; second, ten provinces are located above the 2500 masl; and third, there is a marked inequality among its inhabitants.

The three main ethnic groups are Mestizos, Afro-Ecuadorians and Native Amerindians. (González-Andrade F, 2018a, 2018b). Main spoken languages are Spanish (Castilian) 93% (official), Kichwa 4.1%, other native languages 0.7%, foreign 2.2%. Kichwa and Shuar are official languages for intercultural relations but there are other indigenous languages officially use by indigenous peoples in the areas they inhabit (González-Andrade F, 2007, 2010, 2012).

The first group is the Mestizos, who are descendants of the crossbreeding between Europeans and Native Amerindians, across more than 500 years of miscegenation which began at the 16th century. Today they represent the majority of the population, where 71.9% of them self-identify as mestizos. Besides this, approximately 14 million people are mestizos which only represent 60% of the whole population.

The second group is the Native Amerindians. In Ecuador there are 13 nationalities and 18 Native Amerindian communities, that reside in three out of four regions of the country but mainly in rural areas. The Native Amerindian Nationalities assume an ethnic identity based on their culture, their believes and the history that defines them. The biggest Native Amerindian group is the Kichwa community, which comprises more than 3 million inhabitants, most of them are located at Chimborazo province. The rest native groups comprise around 100 to 8000 individuals, being small groups. Additionally, Kichwa language is the fourth most spoken in the continent. Native communities share historical, economic, political and cultural traditions, they have their own form of social organization as well as their own administration system based in their identity. They have tangible and intangible cultural values that emphasize diversity (González-Andrade F, 2007, 2010, 2012).

The third group is Afro-Ecuadorians, made up of Black people that descended from African slaves. This group live on the Pacific coast of Ecuador, in the provinces of Esmeraldas and Guayas, with a population close to one million individuals. They descend from the African slaves brought by the Spaniards during colonization. In the Andean region of Ecuador, people of African descent reside in "El valle de Chota", in the province of Imbabura. Most of this Afro-Ecuadorian descend from the survivors of stranded slave ships on the north coast of Ecuador, between the 17th- 18th centuries. Also, another important percentage of slaves arrived in the 18th century from Colombia, obtaining freedom after 1860s.

Besides ethnicity, one of the features that characterize Ecuador its the location at high altitude. Thus, data was obtained and classified according to an altitude range between 3264 and 2500 masl (table 3). It also indicates the distribution of cases numbers by the highest cities in Ecuador and the prevalence rate of CHD from 2008 to 2017. According to table 3, the highest city is Mocha located at province of Tungurahua with 3264 masl. The CHD prevalence rate is variable, between the highest cities. This could be due to the National Health System does not cover the whole country, being the largest cities the only ones that offer pediatric cardiology services, and thus may be the reason for indicating the greater amount of CHD. Another interesting finding is that in the highest cities, where the majority of the population is Native American have little access to health programs. Thus, these two factors combined, location and native ethnic origin, could have an effect in etiology of CHD. Even though, no one has established the implications of both factors acting together, Table 3 suggests a correlation.

Table 3. Distribution of cases number by highest cities in Ecuador and prevalence rate of CHD from 2008 to 2017

Average altitude in masl	City	Canton	Province	Cases	LNB	Rate x10000
3264	Mocha	Mocha	Tungurahua	12	552	217.4
3245	Tisaleo	Tisaleo	Tungurahua	5	940	53.2
3200	Cajabamba	Colta	Chimborazo	4	2918	13.7
3160	Pucará	Pucará	Azuay	11	856	128.5
3125	Cañar	Cañar	Cañar	60	5830	102.9
3060	Guamote	Guamote	Chimborazo	14	6363	22.0
3007	El Ángel	Espejo	Carchi	5	1148	43.6
3000	Huaca	San Pedro	Carchi	1	746	13.4
2990	El Tambo	Catamayo	Cañar	7	1370	51.1
2980	Tulcán	Tulcán	Carchi	90	11747	76.6
2960	Quero	Quero	Tungurahua	22	2078	105.9
2947	Pujilí	Pujilí	Cotopaxi	61	8991	67.8
2945	Machachi	Mejia	Pichincha	71	10804	65.7
2920	Saquisilí	Saquisilí	Cotopaxi	11	4492	24.5
2892	Cevallos	Cevallos	Tungurahua	7	774	90.4
2877	Tabacundo	Pedro Moncayo	Pichincha	39	4432	88.0
2870	San Gabriel	Montúfar	Carchi	11	3421	32.2
2864	Nabón	Nabón	Azuay	85	1707	497.9
2850	Quito	Quito	Pichincha	5628	330896	170.1
2830	Cayambe	Cayambe	Pichincha	116	12611	92.0
2800	Píllaro	Santiago	Tungurahua	35	4631	75.6
2764	Riobamba	Riobamba	Chimborazo	355	42369	83.8
2750	Latacunga	Latacunga	Cotopaxi	297	27077	109.7
2740	Guano	Guano	Chimborazo	14	5256	26.6
2720	Suscal	Suscal	Cañar	4	752	53.2
2690	San Fernando	San Fernando	Azuay	0	394	0.0
2683	Salcedo	Salcedo	Cotopaxi	36	8139	44.2
2675	Déleg	Déleg	Cañar	2	454	44.1
2668	Guaranda	Guaranda	Bolívar	101	14791	68.3
2620	Biblián	Biblián	Cañar	20	3201	62.5
2605	Bolívar	Bolívar	Carchi	8	24488	3.3
2600	Pelileo	San Pedro de Pelileo	Tungurahua	30	8484	35.4
2550	Cuenca	Cuenca	Azuay	1063	85671	124.1
2550	Otavalo	Otavalo	Imbabura	133	19142	69.5
2530	Saraguro	Sarguro	Loja	26	4020	64.7
2518	Azogues	Azogues	Cañar	122	12008	101.6
2500	Ambato	Ambato	Tungurahua	462	51579	89.6
2500	Sangolquí	Rumuñahui	Pichincha	127	11371	111.7

LNB = live newborns; rate calculated by 10,000 newborns.
Data source: INEC.
Elaboration and analysis: authors.

According to registries of hospital discharges (INEC, 2019), the number of cases of CHD reported was 34904 cases in 18 years, with a mean of 1939 cases discharged per year. It analyzed the ICD-10 codes Q20 to Q28. The most common CHD by group was Q21, CHD of cardiac septa with 9,620 cases; followed by Q25, CHD of the great arteries with 8585 cases. By specific pathology were Q25.0, patent ductus arteriosus with 6002 cases; Q24.0, dextrocardia with 5175 cases; Q24.9 CHD unspecified, and Q21.0 with 2831 cases. National mean prevalence rate of CHD was 70.63, calculated by 4885 cases in 4′941,073 live newborns. The year that reported more cases were 2013 with a prevalence rate of 97.5 per 10,000 live newborns, followed by 2015, with 94.5 per 10,000 live newborns. Mean prevalence rate was 70.63, calculated by 4885 cases in 4′941,073 live newborns. The year that reported more cases were 2013 with a prevalence rate of 97.5 per 10,000 live newborns, followed by 2015, with 94.5 per 10,000 live newborns. Table 5 shows these results.

Some cities showed in the table are capitals, with greater availability and accessibility of health services. This can be a confounding factor when identifying cases. The records analyzed are from hospital discharges, which this does not allow us to establish if all are unique admissions or also re-admissions. The highest prevalence rate reported in developing countries is 125 per 10000 live newborn, while in Ecuador prevalence rates are between 128.5 to 497.9 cases by 10,000 live newborns, which is a markedly significant fact, and it, which coincides with our hypothesis that high altitudes can increase CHD.

Table 4 shows the number of cases and prevalence rate above the national mean altitude, at 17 locations. This is an interesting finding that deserves to be studied in depth. It could be thought that the higher cities have a higher prevalence rate; however, this could not be affirmed in a restrictive way since many cases are referred to larger health establishments, which accumulate casuistry. It is a fact is that these cities are rural and mostly habited by Native Amerindians.

Table 4. Distribution of number of cases by highest prevalence rate of congenital cardiopathies in Ecuador and average altitude per city from 2008 to 2017

Average altitude in masl	City	Canton	Province	Cases	LNB	Rate x10000
2864	Nabón	Nabón	Azuay	85	1707	**497.9**
3264	Mocha	Mocha	Tungurahua	12	552	**217.4**
2850	Quito	Quito	Pichincha	5628	330896	**170.1**
3160	Pucará	Pucará	Azuay	11	856	**128.5**
2550	Cuenca	Cuenca	Azuay	1063	85671	**124.1**
2750	Latacunga	Latacunga	Cotopaxi	297	27077	**109.7**
2500	Sangolquí	Rumuñahui	Pichincha	127	11371	**111.7**
2960	Quero	Quero	Tungurahua	22	2078	**105.9**
3125	Cañar	Cañar	Cañar	60	5830	**102.9**
2518	Azogues	Azogues	Cañar	122	12008	**101.6**
2830	Cayambe	Cayambe	Pichincha	116	12611	**92.0**
2892	Cevallos	Cevallos	Tungurahua	7	774	**90.4**
2500	Ambato	Ambato	Tungurahua	462	51579	**89.6**
2877	Tabacundo	Pedro Moncayo	Pichincha	39	4432	**88.0**
2764	Riobamba	Riobamba	Chimborazo	355	42369	**83.8**
2980	Tulcán	Tulcán	Carchi	90	11747	**76.6**
2800	Píllaro	Santiago	Tungurahua	35	4631	**75.6**
National mean prevalence rate				34885	4941073	**70.6**
2550	Otavalo	Otavalo	Imbabura	133	19142	**69.5**
2668	Guaranda	Guaranda	Bolívar	101	14791	**68.3**
2947	Pujilí	Pujilí	Cotopaxi	61	8991	**67.8**
2945	Machachi	Mejía	Pichincha	71	10804	**65.7**
2530	Saraguro	Sarguro	Loja	26	4020	**64.7**
2620	Biblián	Biblián	Cañar	20	3201	**62.5**
3245	Tisaleo	Tisaleo	Tungurahua	5	940	**53.2**
2720	Suscal	Suscal	Cañar	4	752	**53.2**
2990	El Tambo	Catamayo	Cañar	7	1370	**51.1**
2683	Salcedo	Salcedo	Cotopaxi	36	8139	**44.2**
2675	Déleg	Déleg	Cañar	2	454	**44.1**
3007	El Ángel	Espejo	Carchi	5	1148	**43.6**
2600	Pelileo	San Pedro	Tungurahua	30	8484	**35.4**
2870	San Gabriel	Montúfar	Carchi	11	3421	**32.2**
2740	Guano	Guano	Chimborazo	14	5256	**26.6**
2920	Saquisilí	Saquisilí	Cotopaxi	11	4492	**24.5**
3060	Guamote	Guamote	Chimborazo	14	6363	**22.0**
3200	Cajabamba	Colta	Chimborazo	4	2918	**13.7**
3000	Huaca	San Pedro	Carchi	1	746	**13.4**
2605	Bolívar	Bolívar	Carchi	8	24488	**3.3**
2690	San Fernando	San Fernando	Azuay	0	394	**0.0**

LNB = live newborns; rate calculated by 10,000 newborns.
Data source: INEC.
Elaboration and analysis: authors.

CONCLUSION

High altitude above 2500 masl, ethnicity (Native American) and rural locations are factors that influence and increase the prevalence rate of CHD. It is a fact that the highest prevalence rate reported in developed countries is 125/10000 LNB, in comparison with Ecuador, that reports higher prevalence rates between 128.5 to 497.9 cases by 10,000 LNB, which is a markedly significant fact, and it coincides with our hypothesis that high altitudes could increase CHD. Other factor important is that higher prevalence rates are seen mostly in locations at rural areas.

In order to answer chronic adaptation questions associated with high altitude exposure, functional experimentation is needed. Identifying epigenetic modifications, gaining insight into the molecular mechanisms of adaptive change in Andean populations as the current knowledge is limited. Such knowledge is important in order to understand biological traits and its genetic control on human patterns, origins, and the evolutionary forces that maintain them. It needs further research.

Note: This manuscript has been openly reviewed by peers, by Mauricio Medina of the Central University of Ecuador and Lorena Rubio of the San Francisco University of Quito, Ecuador.

ANNEX 1

Table 5. Number of cases of congenital diseases of the circulatory system according to hospital discharges, classified according to ICD-10 (Q20-Q28), between 2000 and 2017

	2000	2001	2002	2003	2004	2005	2006	2007	2008	2009	2010	2011	2012	2013	2014	2015	2016	2017	Total
(Q20) Congenital malformations of cardiac chambers and their connections	332	309	429	242	213	175	214	256	258	254	397	365	268	259	268	259	182	200	4909
(Q20.0) Common arterial trunk	5	7	5	2	3	0	10	4	7	16	13	12	9	10	13	13	13	17	159
(Q20.1) Transposition of the great vessels in the right ventricle	1	1	2	22	20	0	2	3	7	6	10	7	2	17	21	20	16	17	174
Q20.2) Transposition of the great vessels in the left ventricle	1	1	3	0	0	0	0	0	2	3	5	1	5	8	4	3	1	8	45
(Q20.3) Discordance of ventricle-arterial connection, transposition of the great vessels	17	32	28	0	0	14	22	18	12	24	30	35	24	32	31	23	26	23	391
(Q20.4) Ventricle with double entry	12	16	18	9	10	16	20	18	15	25	36	20	16	25	21	25	25	34	361
(Q20.5) Discordance of atrio-ventricular connection	292	248	336	203	175	137	148	192	204	166	280	259	186	150	115	113	20	3	3227

Table 5. (Continued)

	2000	2001	2002	2003	2004	2005	2006	2007	2008	2009	2010	2011	2012	2013	2014	2015	2016	2017	Total
(Q20.6) Isomerism of the atrial appendages	0	0	0	0	0	0	0	2	2	1	0	2	1	3	2	1	0	3	17
(Q20.8) Other congenital malformations of cardiac chambers and their connections	1	3	6	1	5	3	8	3	6	4	6	13	8	8	12	15	9	25	136
(Q20.9) Congenital malformation of cardiac chambers and their connections, unspecified	3	1	31	5	0	5	4	16	3	9	17	16	17	35	49	46	72	70	399
(Q21) Congenital malformations of cardiac septa	146	160	271	212	235	246	355	407	472	555	707	810	692	822	781	895	878	976	9620
(Q21.0) Ventricular septum defect	4	21	42	42	71	58	132	107	152	160	207	254	244	291	268	279	221	278	2831
(Q21.1) Atrial septum defect	18	23	42	42	55	57	87	127	123	146	181	241	193	247	226	310	364	308	2790
(Q21.2) Atrio-ventricular septum defect	16	22	39	24	22	23	24	32	40	55	77	71	66	72	66	66	78	92	885
(Q21.3) Fallot tetralogy	103	81	138	95	77	85	94	126	127	111	204	199	146	145	147	142	99	140	2259

	2000	2001	2002	2003	2004	2005	2006	2007	2008	2009	2010	2011	2012	2013	2014	2015	2016	2017	Total
(Q21.4) Aortopulmonary septum defect	2	1	1	2	4	1	3	6	5	10	6	3	3	2	2	1	3	3	58
(Q21.8) Other congenital malformations of cardiac septa	1	6	6	3	3	1	7	5	10	12	7	4	10	16	7	2	8	13	121
(Q21.9) Congenital malformation of cardiac septum, unspecified	2	6	3	4	3	21	8	4	15	61	25	38	30	49	65	95	105	142	676
(Q22) Congenital malformations of the pulmonary and tricuspid valves	34	78	57	93	59	73	124	78	95	91	79	99	89	90	135	174	137	140	1725
(Q22.0) Pulmonary valve atresia	0	7	2	1	0	1	8	11	7	8	5	8	12	12	34	41	28	29	214
(Q22.1) Congenital pulmonary valve stenosis	0	2	0	4	2	2	9	9	4	8	9	8	7	6	5	11	15	12	113
(Q22.2) Congenital pulmonary valve insufficiency	0	1	0	0	0	1	1	0	3	2	0	0	0	0	1	0	0	1	10
(Q22.3) Other congenital malformations of the pulmonary valve	0	2	1	1	4	20	45	2	18	1	4	9	9	7	3	4	5	5	140

Table 5. (Continued)

	2000	2001	2002	2003	2004	2005	2006	2007	2008	2009	2010	2011	2012	2013	2014	2015	2016	2017	Total
(Q22.4) Congenital stenosis of the tricuspid valve	21	31	15	14	18	16	14	18	33	34	25	31	20	20	44	46	33	27	460
(Q22.5) Ebstein's anomaly	9	14	22	19	21	12	23	25	12	19	22	28	26	18	26	42	32	36	406
(Q22.6) Right heart hypoplasia syndrome	0	2	0	0	0	0	5	1	1	0	1	4	2	1	9	7	5	6	44
(Q22.8) Other congenital malformations of the tricuspid valve	4	15	16	54	14	21	18	8	14	17	11	10	11	17	3	14	11	10	268
(Q22.9) Congenital malformation of tricuspid valve, unspecified	0	4	1	0	0	0	1	4	3	2	2	1	2	9	10	9	8	14	70
(Q23) Congenital malformations of the aortic and mitral valves	31	25	41	37	23	23	33	33	26	42	48	40	26	44	37	31	41	43	624
(Q23.0) Congenital stenosis of the aortic valve	16	10	15	22	10	14	5	14	8	16	15	16	2	9	6	8	9	6	201

	2000	2001	2002	2003	2004	2005	2006	2007	2008	2009	2010	2011	2012	2013	2014	2015	2016	2017	Total
(Q22.4) Congenital stenosis of the tricuspid valve	21	31	15	14	18	16	14	18	33	34	25	31	20	20	44	46	33	27	460
(Q23.1) Congenital insufficiency of the aortic valve	6	6	6	3	3	3	7	2	3	4	6	10	5	13	4	2	6	2	91
(Q23.2) Congenital mitral stenosis	0	0	2	4	0	0	2	3	0	2	4	3	4	3	4	3	2	3	39
(Q23.3) Congenital mitral insufficiency	5	2	10	3	3	1	6	6	4	7	13	6	6	6	6	6	5	7	102
(Q23.4) Hypoplastic left heart syndrome	2	1	3	0	2	1	6	3	6	7	6	3	5	7	11	9	14	20	106
(Q23.8) Other congenital malformations of the aortic and mitral valves	1	3	2	1	1	0	3	2	1	1	1	0	1	1	0	0	1	3	22
(Q23.9) Congenital malformation of the aortic and mitral valves, unspecified	1	3	3	4	4	4	4	3	4	5	3	2	3	5	6	3	4	2	63
(Q24) Other congenital heart malformations	282	249	236	283	288	244	293	268	340	289	324	338	326	412	318	249	216	220	5175
(Q24.0) Dextrocardia	0	4	1	4	4	4	8	11	14	11	14	13	14	24	13	18	16	15	188
(Q24.1) Levocardia	1	0	0	0	0	1	0	0	0	0	0	1	1	1	0	1	1	0	7

Table 5. (Continued)

	2000	2001	2002	2003	2004	2005	2006	2007	2008	2009	2010	2011	2012	2013	2014	2015	2016	2017	Total
(Q24.2) Triauricular heart	1	0	0	0	0	0	0	1	0	1	1	2	2	2	0	1	3	1	15
(Q24.3) Pulmonary infundibular stenosis	1	0	3	0	1	3	0	4	1	1	3	0	1	4	6	2	0	2	32
(Q24.4) Congenital subaortic stenosis	0	3	0	0	1	0	2	1	0	1	2	3	5	2	7	2	4	2	35
(Q24.5) Coronary vessel malformation	5	2	3	0	7	2	5	7	5	1	12	16	16	10	12	6	10	3	122
(Q24.6) Congenital heart block	2	0	0	0	1	1	4	2	3	1	1	0	5	34	5	2	5	3	69
(Q24.8) Other congenital heart malformations, specified	32	28	46	46	21	17	70	16	25	28	18	19	19	36	31	42	22	31	547
(Q24.9) Congenital heart malformation, unspecified	240	212	183	233	252	217	204	226	292	245	272	284	263	300	243	175	156	163	4160
(Q25) Congenital malformations of the great arteries	371	359	400	329	343	339	367	409	462	522	562	573	584	574	566	637	597	591	8585
(Q25.0) Patent ductus arteriosus	277	235	283	196	249	237	269	280	335	386	423	399	412	389	397	457	416	362	6002
(Q25.1) Coarctation of the aorta	24	18	31	15	14	31	31	42	29	41	42	47	45	74	68	62	61	96	771

	2000	2001	2002	2003	2004	2005	2006	2007	2008	2009	2010	2011	2012	2013	2014	2015	2016	2017	Total
(Q25.2) Atresia of the aorta	0	0	1	0	0	0	0	0	2	1	0	1	0	2	1	1	1	4	14
(Q25.3) Aortic stenosis	18	22	17	29	28	25	22	19	25	21	27	32	53	30	24	27	25	17	461
(Q25.4) Other congenital malformations of the aorta	9	18	9	5	6	2	4	8	5	0	10	2	5	5	12	8	5	10	123
(Q25.5) Pulmonary artery atresia	9	20	23	27	11	14	21	19	30	26	22	19	20	23	13	25	18	17	357
(Q25.6) Pulmonary artery stenosis	19	22	20	18	10	13	9	23	9	19	17	24	15	15	12	8	10	11	274
(Q25.7) Other congenital malformations of the pulmonary artery	11	12	8	32	0	1	3	5	10	5	3	5	7	6	2	5	2	1	118
(Q25.8) Other congenital malformations of the great arteries	0	0	0	2	3	3	4	4	6	10	7	13	2	4	3	3	3	9	76
(Q25.9) Congenital malformation of the great arteries, unspecified	4	12	8	5	22	13	4	9	11	13	11	31	25	26	34	41	56	64	389
(Q26) Congenital malformations of the great veins	27	24	12	7	5	13	15	19	16	18	16	19	117	51	53	39	33	38	522
(Q26.0) Congenital stenosis of the vena cava	0	0	0	0	0	0	1	0	2	0	1	2	1	0	1	0	1	3	12
(Q26.1) Persistence of the upper left vena cava	0	0	0	0	0	1	0	0	1	0	0	1	0	0	1	1	0	1	7

Table 5. (Continued)

	2000	2001	2002	2003	2004	2005	2006	2007	2008	2009	2010	2011	2012	2013	2014	2015	2016	2017	Total
(Q26.2) Total anomalous connection of the pulmonary veins	0	1	1	2	1	2	0	1	1	2	0	0	4	17	21	15	10	13	91
(Q26.3) Partial anomalous connection of the pulmonary veins	0	0	0	0	0	1	0	3	0	0	2	0	1	2	1	2	5	1	18
(Q26.4) Abnormal connection of the pulmonary veins, without other specification	21	18	7	3	3	4	6	7	4	8	7	8	12	12	4	4	3	7	138
(Q26.5) Abnormal connection of the portal vein	0	0	0	0	0	1	0	0	1	1	0	0	0	0	2	0	0	3	8
(Q26.6) Fistula hepatic artery-portal vein	3	1	4	0	0	2	3	2	4	1	0	1	8	2	4	1	1	0	37
(Q26.8) Other congenital malformations of the great veins	0	0	0	0	0	0	4	1	2	5	1	5	81	13	8	8	5	5	138
(Q26.9) Congenital malformation of large veins, unspecified	3	4	0	2	1	2	1	5	1	1	5	2	9	5	11	8	8	5	73
(Q27) Other congenital malformations of the peripheral vascular system	24	28	36	28	20	26	21	20	22	32	31	57	79	103	49	48	58	71	753

	2000	2001	2002	2003	2004	2005	2006	2007	2008	2009	2010	2011	2012	2013	2014	2015	2016	2017	Total
(Q27.0) Absence and congenital hypoplasia of the umbilical artery	0	2	0	1	0	2	0	2	0	2	1	0	3	4	1	1	1	2	22
(Q27.1) Congenital renal artery stenosis	0	1	1	0	0	0	0	0	2	1	0	6	2	3	2	1	1	0	20
(Q27.2) Other congenital malformations of the renal artery	0	0	0	0	1	0	0	0	0	1	1	0	0	1	0	1	0	0	5
(Q27.3) Peripheral arteriovenous malformation	5	9	7	5	4	6	7	1	1	11	11	14	36	46	15	28	38	40	284
(Q27.4) Congenital phlebectasia	0	0	0	0	0	0	0	0	0	0	0	0	0	0	0	0	0	2	2
(Q27.8) Other congenital malformations of the peripheral vascular system, specified	3	1	4	8	0	5	3	4	7	3	6	11	12	12	14	5	7	8	113
(Q27.9) Congenital malformation of the peripheral	16	15	24	14	15	13	11	13	12	14	12	26	26	37	17	12	11	19	307

Table 5. (Continued)

	2000	2001	2002	2003	2004	2005	2006	2007	2008	2009	2010	2011	2012	2013	2014	2015	2016	2017	Total
vascular system, unspecified																			
(Q28) Other congenital malformations of the circulatory system	41	41	52	50	65	50	79	69	110	126	148	205	272	317	292	345	386	332	2980
(Q28.0) Arteriovenous malformation of precerebral vessels	0	1	0	0	1	2	1	1	1	5	5	12	5	21	14	8	16	13	106
(Q28.1) Other malformations of precerebral vessels	0	0	0	2	0	1	3	0	2	0	0	0	0	3	1	0	2	1	15
(Q28.2) Arteriovenous malformation of cerebral vessels	27	35	40	35	46	38	63	53	84	106	113	166	235	245	249	294	325	265	2419
(Q28.3) Other malformations of the cerebral vessels	13	4	11	10	9	6	9	11	15	11	19	14	14	15	14	17	8	27	227
(Q28.8) Other congenital malformations of the circulatory system, specified	0	0	0	0	8	1	3	1	3	1	3	1	1	4	9	7	5	5	52

	2000	2001	2002	2003	2004	2005	2006	2007	2008	2009	2010	2011	2012	2013	2014	2015	2016	2017	Total
vascular system, unspecified																			
(Q28) Other congenital malformations of the circulatory system	41	41	52	50	65	50	79	69	110	126	148	205	272	317	292	345	386	332	2980
(Q28.0) Arteriovenous malformation of precerebral vessels	0	1	0	0	1	2	1	1	1	5	5	12	5	21	14	8	16	13	106
(Q28.1) Other malformations of precerebral vessels	0	0	0	2	0	1	3	0	2	0	0	0	0	3	1	0	2	1	15
(Q28.9) Congenital malformation of the circulatory system, unspecified	1	1	1	3	1	2	0	3	5	3	8	12	17	29	5	19	30	21	161
Total	2611	2529	2677	2502	2708	2453	2506	2312	1929	1801	1559	1501	1189	1251	1281	1534	1273	1288	**34904**

REFERENCES

Appenzeller, Otto, Tamara Minko, Clifford Qualls, Vitaly Pozharov, Jorge Gamboa, Alfredo Gamboa, and Yang Wang. 2006. "Gene Expression, Autonomic Function and Chronic Hypoxia: Lessons from the Andes." *Clinical Autonomic Research* 16 (3): 217–22. https://doi.org/10.1007/s10286-006-0338-3.

Arias, J., and M. Topilsky. 1971. "Anatomy of the Coronary Circulation at High Altitude." *High Altitude Physiology Cardiac and Respiratory Aspects*, no. 6: 149–54. https://doi.org/10.1152/jappl.1983.55.6.1942.

Bajolle, Fanny, Stéphane Zaffran, and Damien Bonnet. 2009. "Genetics and Embryological Mechanisms of Congenital Heart Diseases." *Archives of Cardiovascular Diseases* 102 (1): 59–63. https://doi.org/10.1016/j.acvd.2008.06.020.

Beall, Cynthia. 2000. "Tibetan and Andean Contrasts in Adaptation to High-Altitude Hypoxia." *Advances in Experimental Medicine and Biology* 475 (1): 63–74. http://www.ncbi.nlm.nih.gov/pubmed/10849649.

——— . 2007. "Two Routes to Functional Adaptation: Tibetan and Andean High-Altitude Natives." *Proceedings of the National Academy of Sciences of the United States of America* 104 (1): 8655–60. https://doi.org/10.1111/j.1550-7408.1980.tb05388.x.

Beall, Cynthia M., Daniel Laskowski, and Serpil C. Erzurum. 2012. "Nitric Oxide in Adaptation to Altitude." *Free Radical Biology and Medicine* 52 (7): 1123–34. https://doi.org/10.1016/j.freeradbiomed.2011.12.028.

Bhagi, Shuchi, Swati Srivastava, Arvind Tomar, Shashi Bala Singh, and Soma Sarkar. 2015. "Positive Association of D Allele of ACE Gene With High Altitude Pulmonary Edema in Indian Population." *Wilderness and Environmental Medicine* 26 (2): 124–32. https://doi.org/10.1016/j.wem.2014.09.010.

Bigham, Abigail, Marc Bauchet, Dalila Pinto, Xianyun Mao, Joshua M. Akey, Rui Mei, Stephen W. Scherer, et al. 2010. "Identifying Signatures of Natural Selection in Tibetan and Andean Populations Using Dense Genome Scan Data." *PLoS Genetics* 6 (9). https://doi.org/10.1371/journal.pgen.1001116.

Bigham, Abigail W., Xianyun Mao, Rui Mei, Tom Brutsaert, Megan J. Wilson, Colleen Glyde Julian, Esteban J. Parra, Joshua M. Akey, Lorna G. Moore, and Mark D. Shriver. 2009. "Identifying Positive Selection Candidate Loci for High-Altitude Adaptation in Andean Populations." *Human Genomics* 4 (2): 79–90. http://www.ncbi.nlm.nih.gov/pubmed/20038496%0Ahttp://www.pubmedcentral.nih.gov/articlerender.fcgi?artid=PMC2857381.

Bigham, Abigail, Megan Wilson, Colleen Julian, Melisa Kiyamu, Enrique Vargas, Fabiola Leon-Velarde, Maria Rivera-Chira, et al. 2013. "Andean and Tibetan Patterns of Adaptation to High Altitude." *American Journal of Human Biology* 25 (2): 190–97. https://doi.org/10.1002/ajhb.22358.

Brown, James P. R., and Michael P. W. Grocott. 2013. "Humans at Altitude: Physiology and Pathophysiology." *Continuing Education in Anaesthesia, Critical Care and Pain* 13 (1): 17–22. https://doi.org/10.1093/bjaceaccp/mks047.

Cangussú, Luana Resende, Matheus Rodrigues Lopes, and Romero Henrique de Almeida Barbosa. 2019. "The Importance of the Early Diagnosis of Aorta Coarctation." *Revista Da Associação Médica Brasileira* 65 (2): 240–45. https://doi.org/10.1590/1806-9282.65.2.240.

Chiodi, Hugo. 1957. *"Respiratory Adaptations to Chronic High Altitude Hypoxia."* American Physiological Society.

Choi, Eun Hwa, Mary Ehrmantraut, Charles B. Foster, Joel Moss, and Stephen J. Chanock. 2006. "Association of Common Haplotypes of Surfactant Protein A1 and A2 (SFTPA1 and SFTPA2) Genes with Severity of Lung Disease in Cystic Fibrosis." *Pediatric Pulmonology* 41 (3): 255–62. https://doi.org/10.1002/ppul.20361.

Chowdhury, Devyani. 2009. "Pathophysiology of Congenital Heart Diseases." *Annals of Cardiac Anaesthesia* 10 (1): 19. https://doi.org/10.4103/0971-9784.37920.

Chun, Hua, Yan Yue, Yibin Wang, Zhaxi Dawa, Pu Zhen, Qu La, Yang Zong, Yi Qu, and Dezhi Mu. 2018. "High Prevalence of Congenital Heart Disease at High Altitudes in Tibet." *European Journal of*

Preventive Cardiology, 1–4. https://doi.org/10.1177/2047487318812502.

Crawford, Jacob E., Ricardo Amaru, Jihyun Song, Colleen G Julian, Fernando Racimo, A Lima, Jerome I Rotter, et al. 2017. *"Natural Selection on Genes Related to Cardiovascular Health in High-Altitude Adapted Andeans,"* 752–67. https://doi.org/10.1016/j.ajhg.2017.09.023.

Danial, N. N. 2008. "Bad: Undertaker by Night, Candyman by Day." *Oncogene* 27 (SUPPL. 1): S53–70. https://doi.org/10.1038/onc.2009.44.

Digilio, M. C., F. Pugnaloni, A. De Luca, G. Calcagni, A. Baban, M. L. Dentici, P. Versacci, B. Dallapiccola, M. Tartaglia, and B. Marino. 2019. "Atrioventricular Canal Defect and Genetic Syndromes: The Unifying Role of Sonic Hedgehog." *Clinical Genetics* 95 (2): 268–76. https://doi.org/10.1111/cge.13375.

Dunham-Snary, Kimberly J., Danchen Wu, Edward A. Sykes, Amar Thakrar, Leah R. G. Parlow, Jeffrey D. Mewburn, Joel L. Parlow, and Stephen L. Archer. 2017. "Hypoxic Pulmonary Vasoconstriction: From Molecular Mechanisms to Medicine." *Chest* 151 (1): 181–92. https://doi.org/10.1016/j.chest.2016.09.001.

Dunwoodie, Sally L. 2007. "Combinatorial Signaling in the Heart Orchestrates Cardiac Induction, Lineage Specification and Chamber Formation." *Seminars in Cell and Developmental Biology* 18 (1): 54–66. https://doi.org/10.1016/j.semcdb.2006.12.003.

Eichstaedt, Christina A., Tiago Antão, Luca Pagani, Alexia Cardona, Toomas Kivisild, and Maru Mormina. 2014. "The Andean Adaptive Toolkit to Counteract High Altitude Maladaptation: Genome-Wide and Phenotypic Analysis of the Collas." *PLoS ONE* 9 (3). https://doi.org/10.1371/journal.pone.0093314.

Favier, F. B., F. A. Britto, D. G. Freyssenet, X. A. Bigard, and H. Benoit. 2015. "HIF-1-Driven Skeletal Muscle Adaptations to Chronic Hypoxia: Molecular Insights into Muscle Physiology." *Cellular and Molecular Life Sciences* 72 (24): 4681–96. https://doi.org/10.1007/s00018-015-2025-9.

Fluck, M. 2006. "Functional, Structural and Molecular Plasticity of Mammalian Skeletal Muscle in Response to Exercise Stimuli." *Journal of Experimental Biology* 209 (12): 2239–48. https://doi.org/10.1242/jeb.02149.

Forsey, Jonathan T., Ola A. Elmasry, and Robin P. Martin. 2009. "Patent Arterial Duct." *Orphanet Journal of Rare Diseases* 4 (1): 1–9. https://doi.org/10.1186/1750-1172-4-17.

Freeze, Samantha L., Benjamin J. Landis, Stephanie M. Ware, and Benjamin M. Helm. 2016. "Bicuspid Aortic Valve: A Review with Recommendations for Genetic Counseling." *Journal of Genetic Counseling* 25 (6): 1171–78. https://doi.org/10.1007/s10897-016-0002-6.

Frisancho, A. Roberto. 2013. "Developmental Functional Adaptation to High Altitude: Review." American Journal of Human Biology 25 (2): 151–68. https://doi.org/10.1002/ajhb.22367.

Gao, Yuansheng, and J. Raj. 2009. "Endothelial Regulation of the Pulmonary Circulation in the Fetus and Newborn." *The Pulmonary Endothelium: Function in Health and Disease,* no. 258: 379–97. https://doi.org/10.1002/9780470747490.ch23.

García, Alberto, Karen Moreno, Miguel Ronderos, Néstor Sandoval, Mónica Caicedo, and Rodolfo J. Dennis. 2016. "Differences by Altitude in the Frequency of Congenital Heart Defects in Colombia." *Pediatric Cardiology* 37 (8): 1507–15. https://doi.org/10.1007/s00246-016-1464-x.

Gassmann, Norina N., Hugo A. van Elteren, Tom G. Goos, Claudia R. Morales, Maria Rivera-Ch, Daniel S. Martin, Patricia Cabala Peralta, et al. 2016. "Pregnancy at High Altitude in the Andes Leads to Increased Total Vessel Density in Healthy Newborns." *Journal of Applied Physiology* 121 (3): 709–15. https://doi.org/10.1152/japplphysiol.00561.2016.

Gerich, John E., Christian Meyer, Hans J. Woerle, and Michael Stumvoll. 1963. "Renal Gluconeogenesis." *Advances in Enzyme Regulation* 24 (2). https://doi.org/10.1016/0065-2571(63)90034-7.

Gilbert-Kawai, Edward T., James S. Milledge, Michael P.W. Grocott, and Daniel S. Martin. 2014. "King of the Mountains: Tibetan and Sherpa Physiological Adaptations for Life at High Altitude." *Physiology* 29 (6): 388–402. https://doi.org/10.1152/physiol.00018.2014.

Gonzales, Gustavo F. 2012. "[Impact of High Altitude on Pregnancy and Newborn Parameters]." *Revista Peruana de Medicina Experimental y Salud Publica* 29 (2): 242–49.

Gonzales, Gustavo F., Dulce E. Alarcón-Yaquetto, and Alisson Zevallos-Concha. 2016. "Human Adaptation to Life at High Altitude." In *Biochemistry of Oxidative Stress: Physiopathology and Clinical Aspects,* edited by Ricardo Jorge Gelpi, Alberto Boveris, and Juan José Poderoso, 109–26. Cham: Springer International Publishing. https://doi.org/10.1007/978-3-319-45865-6_8.

González-Andrade F., Echeverría D., López V., Arellano M. 2018a "Is pulse oximetry helpful for the early detection of critical congenital heart disease at high altitude?" *Congenit Heart Dis.* 13(6):911-918. doi: 10.1111/chd.12654.

González-Andrade F. "Standardized clinical criteria and sweat test combined as a tool to diagnose Cystic Fibrosis". *Heliyon.* 2018b Dec 17;4(12):e01050. doi: 10.1016/j.heliyon.2018.e01050. eCollection 2018 Dec.

González-Andrade F., López-Pulles R. "Congenital malformations in Ecuadorian children: urgent need to create a National Registry of Birth Defects". *2012. Appl Clin Genet.* 14;3:29-39. doi: https://doi.org/10.2147/TACG.S8794.

González-Andrade F., López-Pulles R. "Ecuador: public health genomics". 2010. *Public Health Genomics.* 13(3):171-80. doi: 10.1159/000249817.

González-Andrade F., Sánchez D., González-Solórzano J., Gascón S., Martínez-Jarreta B. "Sex-specific genetic admixture of Mestizos, Amerindian Kichwas, and Afro-Ecuadorans from Ecuador." 2007. *Hum Biol.* 79(1):51-77.

Graves, Barbara W., and Mary Mumford Haley. 2013. "Newborn Transition." *Journal of Midwifery and Women's Health* 58 (6): 662–70. https://doi.org/10.1111/jmwh.12097.

Grocott, Michael, Hugh Montgomery, and Andre Vercueil. 2007. "High-Altitude Physiology and Pathophysiology: Implications and Relevance for Intensive Care Medicine." *Critical Care* 11 (1): 1–5. https://doi.org/10.1186/cc5142.

Gruber, Peter J., and Jonathan A. Epstein. 2004. "Development Gone Awry: Congenital Heart Disease." *Circulation Research* 94 (3): 273–83. https://doi.org/10.1161/01.RES.0000116144.43797.3B.

Guillemin, Karen, and Mark A. Krasnow. 1997. "The Hypoxic Response: Huffing and HIFing." *Cell* 89 (1): 9–12. https://doi.org/10.1016/S0092-8674(00)80176-2.

Hagberg, Carolina E., Annelie Falkevall, Xun Wang, Erik Larsson, Jenni Huusko, Ingrid Nilsson, Laurens A. Van Meeteren, et al. 2010. "Vascular Endothelial Growth Factor B Controls Endothelial Fatty Acid Uptake." *Nature* 464 (7290): 917–21. https://doi.org/10.1038/natu re08 945.

Hasan, Asif. 2016. "Relationship of High Altitude and Congenital Heart Disease." *Indian Heart Journal* 68 (1): 9–12. https://doi.org/10.1016/j.ihj.2015.12.015.

Heinrich, Erica C., Lu Wu, Elijah S. Lawrence, Amy M. Cole, Cecilia Anza-Ramirez, Francisco C. Villafuerte, and Tatum S. Simonson. 2019. "Genetic Variants at the EGLN1 Locus Associated with High-Altitude Adaptation in Tibetans Are Absent or Found at Low Frequency in Highland Andeans." *Annals of Human Genetics* 83 (3): 171–76. https://doi.org/10.1111/ahg.12299.

Hillman, Noah H., Suhas G Kallapur, and Alan H. Jobe. 2012. "Physiology of Transition from Intrauterine to Extrauterine Life." *Clinics in Perinatology* 39 (4): 769–83. https://doi.org/10.1016/j.clp.2012.09.009.

Hochachka, Peter W., and Jim L. Rupert. 2003. "Fine Tuning the HIF-1 'global' O2 Sensor for Hypobaric Hypoxia in Andean High-Altitude Natives." *BioEssays* 25 (5): 515–19. https://doi.org/10.1002/bies.10261.

Holden, J. E., C. K. Stone, C. M. Clark, W. D. Brown, R. J. Nickles, C. Stanley, and P. W. Hochachka. 1995. "Enhanced Cardiac Metabolism of Plasma Glucose in High-Altitude Natives: Adaptation against Chronic Hypoxia." *Journal of Applied Physiology* 79 (1): 222–28. https://doi.org/10.1152/jappl.1995.79.1.222.

Hoppeler, H., E. Kleinert, C. Schlegel, H. Claassen, H. Howald, S. Kayar, and P. Cerretelli. 1990. "II. Morphological Adaptations of Human Skeletal Muscle to Chronic Hypoxia." *International Journal of Sports Medicine* 11 (S 1): S3–9. https://doi.org/10.1055/s-2007-1024846.

Huang, Jing B., Ying Long Liu, and Xiao Dong Lv. 2010. "Pathogenic Mechanisms of Congenital Heart Disease." *Fetal and Pediatric Pathology* 29 (5): 359–72. https://doi.org/10.3109/1551381100 3789628.

Hurtado, Abdias, Elizabeth Escudero, Jackeline Pando, Shailendra Sharma, and Richard J. Johnson. 2012. "Cardiovascular and Renal Effects of Chronic Exposure to High Altitude." *Nephrology Dialysis Transplantation* 27 (SUPPL.4): 11–16. https://doi.org/10.1093/ndt/gfs 427.

INEC. *National Institute of Statistics and Census.* https://www.ecuadoren cifras.gob.ec/estadisticas/.

Iwashima, Satoru, Eichirou Satake, Hiroki Uchiyama, Keigo Seki, and Takamichi Ishikawa. 2018. "Closure Time of Ductus Arteriosus after Birth Based on Survival Analysis." *Early Human Development* 121 (April): 37–43. https://doi.org/10.1016/j.earlhumdev.2018.05.003.

Jacovas, Vanessa Cristina, Diego Luiz Rovaris, Orlando Peréz, Soledad De Azevedo, Gabriel Souza Macedo, José Raul Sandoval, Alberto Salazar-Granara, et al. 2015. "Genetic Variations in the TP53 Pathway in Native Americans Strongly Suggest Adaptation to the High Altitudes of the Andes." *PLoS ONE* 10 (9): 1–15. https://doi.org/10.1371/journal.pone. 0137823.

Jansen, Gerard F. A., Anne Krins, Buddha Basnyat, Joseph A. Odoom, and Can Ince. 2007. "Role of the Altitude Level on Cerebral Autoregulation in Residents at High Altitude." *Journal of Applied Physiology* 103 (2): 518–23. https://doi.org/10.1152/japplphysiol.01429.2006.

Jansen, Gerard F. A., and Buddha Basnyat. 2011. "Brain Blood Flow in Andean and Himalayan High-Altitude Populations: Evidence of Different Traits for the Same Environmental Constraint." *Journal of Cerebral Blood Flow and Metabolism* 31 (2): 706–14. https://doi.org/10.1038/jcbfm.2010.150.

Jefferson, J. Ashley, Jan Simoni, Elizabeth Escudero, Maria-Elena Hurtado, Erik R. Swenson, Donald E. Wesson, George F. Schreiner, Robert B. Schoene, Richard J. Johnson, and Abdias Hurtado. 2004. "Increased Oxidative Stress Following Acute and Chronic High Altitude Exposure." *High Altitude Medicine & Biology* 5 (1): 61–69. https://doi.org/10.1089/152702904322963690.

Julian, Colleen G., and Lorna G. Moore. 2019a. "Human Genetic Adaptation to High Altitude: Evidence from the Andes." *Genes* 10 (2). https://doi.org/10.3390/genes10020150.

———. 2019b. "Human Genetic Adaptation to High Altitude: Evidence from the Andes." *Genes* 10 (2): 1–20. https://doi.org/10.3390/genes10020150.

Julian, Colleen Glyde. 2011. "High Altitude During Pregnancy." *Clinics in Chest Medicine* 32 (1): 21–31. https://doi.org/10.1016/j.ccm.2010.10.008.

Karl, Tom R., and Christian Stocker. 2016. "Tetralogy of Fallot and Its Variants." *Pediatric Critical Care Medicine* 17 (8): S330–36. https://doi.org/10.1097/PCC.0000000000000831.

Kemp, B. E., D. Stapleton, D. J. Campbell, Z.-P. Chen, S Murthy, M. Walter, A. Gupta, et al. 2003. "AMP-Activated Protein Kinase, Super Metabolic Regulator." *Biochemical Society Transactions* 31 (Pt 1): 162–68. https://doi.org/10.1042/.

Kim, John, Merlin Ariefdjohan, Marci Sontag, and Christopher Rausch. 2018. "Pulse Oximetry Values in Newborns with Critical Congenital Heart Disease upon ICU Admission at Altitude." *International Journal of Neonatal Screening* 4 (4): 30. https://doi.org/10.3390/ijns4040030.

Kloesel, Benjamin, James A. DiNardo, and Simon C. Body. 2016. "Cardiac Embryology and Molecular Mechanisms of Congenital Heart Disease."

Anesthesia & Analgesia 123 (3): 551–69. https://doi.org/10.1213/ane. 0000000000001451.

Krock, Bryan L., Nicolas Skuli, and M. Celeste Simon. 2011. "Hypoxia-Induced Angiogenesis: Good and Evil." *Genes and Cancer* 2 (12): 1117–33. https://doi.org/10.1177/1947601911423654.

Li, Jing Jing, Yuan Liu, Si Yuan Xie, Guo Dong Zhao, Ting Dai, Hong Chen, Lan Fang Mu, Hai Ying Qi, and Jia Li. 2019. "Newborn Screening for Congenital Heart Disease Using Echocardiography and Follow-up at High Altitude in China." *International Journal of Cardiology* 274 (xxxx): 106–12. https://doi.org/10.1016/j.ijcard.201 8.08.102.

Li, Shengli, Huaxuan Wen, Meiling Liang, Dandan Luo, Yue Qin, Yimei Liao, Shuyuan Ouyang, et al. 2019. "Congenital Abnormalities of the Aortic Arch: Revisiting the 1964 Stewart Classification." *Cardiovascular Pathology* 39: 38–50. https://doi.org/10.1016/j.carpath.2018. 11.004.

Lozano, Christine M. Eischen and Guillermina. 2016. *"The Mdm Network and Its Regulation of P53 Activities: A Rheostat of Cancer Risk"* 35 (6): 728–37. https://doi.org/10.1002/humu.22524.The.

Luks, Andrew M., Richard J. Johnson, and Erik R. Swenson. 2008. "Chronic Kidney Disease at High Altitude." *Journal of the American Society of Nephrology* 19 (12): 2262–71. https://doi.org/10.1681/asn.2007111199.

Lundby, Carsten, Mikael Sander, Gerrit van Hall, Bengt Saltin, and José A. L. Calbet. 2006. "Maximal Exercise and Muscle Oxygen Extraction in Acclimatizing Lowlanders and High Altitude Natives." *Journal of Physiology* 573 (2): 535–47. https://doi.org/10.1113/jphysiol.2006. 106765.

Merino, Cesar. 2009. "Studies on Blood Formation and Destruction in the Polycythemia of High Altitude." *The Journal of Hematology* 88 (82): 3259–87.

Mitri, Joanna, and Anastassios Pittas. 2014. *"NIH Public Access"* 43 (1): 205–32. https://doi.org/10.1039/b800799c.O.

Moore, Lorna G. 2001. "Human Genetic Adaptation to High Altitude." *High Altitude Medicine & Biology* 2 (2): 257–79.

Mordi, Ify, and Nikolaos Tzemos. 2012. "Bicuspid Aortic Valve Disease: A Comprehensive Review." *Cardiology Research and Practice* 1 (1). Https://doi.org/10.1155/2012/196037.

Moret, P. NR. 1971. "Coronary Blood Flow and Myocardial Metabolism in Man at High Altitude." In *High Altitude Physiology Cardiac and Respiratory Aspects,* 55:131–44. https://doi.org/10.1152/jappl.1983.55.6.1942.

Morton, Sarah U., and Dara Brodsky. 2016. "Fetal Physiology and the Transition to Extrauterine Life." *Clinics in Perinatology* 43 (3): 395–407. https://doi.org/10.1016/j.clp.2016.04.001.

Murray, Andrew J., and James A. Horscroft. 2016. "Mitochondrial Function at Extreme High Altitude." *Journal of Physiology* 594 (5): 1137–49. https://doi.org/10.1113/JP270079.

Niermeyer, Susan. 2003. "Cardiopulmonary Transition in the High Altitude Infant." *High Altitude Medicine & Biology* 4 (2): 225–39. https://doi.org/10.1089/152702903322022820.

Pajuelo, Jaime, José Sánchez, and Hugo Arbañil. 2010. "Las Enfermedades Crónicas No Transmisibles En El Perú y Su Relación Con La Altitud." *Rev Soc Peru Med Interna* 23 (2): 41–80. http://www.sociedadperuanademedicinainterna.org/revista/revista_23_3_2010/revista_spmi_2010_n3.pdf.

Pak, O., A. Aldashev, D. Welsh, and A. Peacock. 2007. "The Effects of Hypoxia On-the Cells of the Pulmonary Vasculature." *European Respiratory Journal* 30 (2): 364–72. https://doi.org/10.1183/09031936.00128706.

Paralikar, Swapnil J., and Jagdish H. Paralikar. 2010. "High-Altitude Medicine." *Indian Journal of Occupational and Environmental Medicina* 14 (1): 6–12. https://doi.org/10.1016/j.mcna.2015.09.002.

Paranka, Michael S., Jeffrey M. Brown, Robert D. White, Matthew V. Park, Amy S. Kelleher, and Reese H. Clark. 2018. "The Impact of Altitude on Screening for Critical Congenital Heart Disease." *Journal of Perinatology* 38 (5): 530–36. https://doi.org/10.1038/s41372-018-0043-9.

Penaloza, Dante, and Javier Arias-Stella. 2007. "The Heart and Pulmonary Circulation at High Altitudes." *Circulation* 115 (9): 1132–46. https://doi.org/10.1161/circulationaha.106.624544.

Picón-Reátegui, E. 1961. "Basal Metabolic Rate and Body Composition at High Altitudes." *Journal of Applied Physiology* 16 (3): 431–34. https://doi.org/10.1152/jappl.1961.16.3.431.

Postigo, Lucrecia, Gladys Heredia, Nicholas P. Illsley, Tatiana Torricos, Caitlin Dolan, Lourdes Echalar, Wilma Tellez, et al. 2009. "Where the O2 Goes to: Preservation of Human Fetal Oxygen Delivery and Consumption at High Altitude." *Journal of Physiology* 587 (3): 693–708. https://doi.org/10.1113/jphysiol.2008.163634.

Priya, Sarv, R. Thomas, P. Nagpal, A. Sharma, and M. Steigner. 2018. "Congenital Anomalies of the Aortic Arch." *Cardiovascular Diagnosis and Therapy* 8 (Suppl 1): s26–44. https://doi.org/10.1007/978-3-319-44691-2_23.

Qaid, Mohammed M., and Mutassim M. Abdelrahman. 2016. "Role of Insulin and Other Related Hormones in Energy Metabolism: A Review." *Cogent Food & Agriculture* 2 (1): 1–18. https://doi.org/10.1080/23311932.2016.1267691.

Reynafarje, Baltazar. 1961. "Myoglobin Content and Enzymatic Activity of Muscle and Altitude Adaptation." *Journal of Applied Physiology* 17 (2): 301–5. https://doi.org/10.1152/jappl.1962.17.2.301.

Roeleveld, Peter P., David M. Axelrod, Darren Klugman, Melissa B. Jones, Nikhil K. Chanani, Joseph W. Rossano, and John M. Costello. 2018. "Hypoplastic Left Heart Syndrome: From Fetus to Fontan." *Cardiology in the Young* 28 (11): 1275–88. https://doi.org/10.1017/s10479511 1800135x.

Sandridge, Amy L., William Greer, Maha Al-Menieir, and Abdullah Al Rowais. 2011. "Exploring the Impact of Altitude on Congenital Heart Defects in Saudi Arabia." *Avicenna*, no. 2010: 3. https://doi.o rg/10.5 339/avi.2010.3.

Shao, Xuesi M. 2019. "High Altitude Exposure during Pregnancy Enhances the Vulnerability of Fetal Heart Dysfunction to Ischemic Stress:

Epigenetic Mechanisms." *International Journal of Cardiology* 274 (xxxx): 59–60. https://doi.org/10.1016/j.ijcard.2018.09.053.

Shiraishi, Isao, and Hajime Ichikawa. 2012. "Human Heterotaxy Syndrome - From Molecular Genetics to Clinical Features, Management, and Prognosis." *Circulation Journal* 76 (9): 2066–75. https://doi.org/10.1253/circj.CJ-12-0957.

Shriver, Mark D., Rui Mei, Abigail Bigham, Xianyun Mao, Tom D. Brutsaert, Esteban J. Parra, and Lorna G. Moore. 2006. "Finding the Genes Underlying Adaptation to Hypoxia Using Genomic Scans for Genetic Adaptation and Admixture Mapping Article." *Advances in Experimental Medicine and Biology* 588 (October 2017). https://doi.org/10.1007/978-0-387-34817-9.

Simha, Vinaya, Muhammad Mahmood, Mohammmed Ansari, Craig W. Spellman, and Pankaj Shah. 2016. "Effect of Vitamin D Replacement on Insulin Sensitivity in Subjects With Vitamin D Deficiency." *Journal of Investigative Medicine* 60 (8): 1214–18. https://doi.org/10.2310/jim.0b013e3182747c06.

Staehr, Peter, Ole Hother-Nielsen, Bernard R. Landau, Visvanathan Chandramouli, Jens Juul Holst, and Henning Beck-nielsen. 2003. "Effects of Free Fatty Acids Per Se on Glucose." *Diabetes* 52 (February): 260–67. http://diabetes.diabetesjournals.org/content/52/2/260.abstract.

Stream, Joshua O., Andrew M. Luks, and Colin K. Grissom. 2009. "Lung Disease at High Altitude." *Expert Review of Respiratory Medicine* 3 (6): 635–50. https://doi.org/10.1586/ers.09.51.

Swanson, Jonathan R., and Robert A. Sinkin. 2015. "Transition from Fetus to Newborn." *Pediatric Clinics of North America* 62 (2): 329–43. https://doi.org/10.1016/j.pcl.2014.11.002.

Swenson, Erik R., and Peter Bärtsch. 2013. "Renal Function and Fluid Homeostasis." *High Altitude* 9781461487: 1–496. https://doi.org/10.1007/978-1-4614-8772-2.

Tin, Win, and Mithilesh Lal. 2015. "Principles of Pulse Oximetry and Its Clinical Application in Neonatal Medicine." *Seminars in Fetal and*

Neonatal Medicine 20 (3): 192–97. https://doi.org/10.1016/j.siny.2015.01.006.

Tomar, Arvind, Seema Malhotra, and Soma Sarkar. 2015. "Polymorphism Profiling of Nine High Altitude Relevant Candidate Gene Loci in Acclimatized Sojourners and Adapted Natives." *BMC Genetics* 16 (1). https://doi.org/10.1186/s12863-015-0268-y.

Vallecilla, Carolina, Reza H. Khiabani, Néstor Sandoval, Mark Fogel, Juan Carlos Briceño, and Ajit P. Yoganathan. 2014. "Effect of High Altitude Exposure on the Hemodynamics of the Bidirectional Glenn Physiology: Modeling Incremented Pulmonary Vascular Resistance and Heart Rate." *Journal of Biomechanics* 47 (8): 1846–52. https://doi.org/10.1016/j.jbiomech.2014.03.021.

Valverde, Guido, Hang Zhou, Sebastian Lippold, Cesare De Filippo, Kun Tang, David López Herráez, Jing Li, and Mark Stoneking. 2015. "A Novel Candidate Region for Genetic Adaptation to High Altitude in Andean Populations." *PLoS ONE* 10 (5): 1–22. https://doi.org/10.1371/journal.pone.0125444.

Vargas, Olga. 2014. *"Exercise and Training at Altitudes : Physiological Effects and Protocols"* 12 (1): 111–26.

Vásquez, René, and Mercedes Villena. 2002. "Normal Hematological Values for Healthy Persons Living at 4000 Meters in Bolivia." *High Altitude Medicine & Biology* 2 (3): 361–67. https://doi.org/10.1089/15270290152608534.

Vogel, J. A., L. H. Hartley, and J. C. Cruz. 1974. "Cardiac Output during Exercise in Altitude Natives at Sea Level and High Altitude." *Journal of Applied Physiology* 36 (2): 173–76. https://doi.org/10.1152/jappl.1974.36.2.173.

Webb, Joanna, Lucinda Perkins, and Malini Ketty. 2016. "Resuscitation of the Term and Preterm Infant." *Paediatrics and Child Health* (United Kingdom) 26 (4): 140–46. https://doi.org/10.1016/j.paed.2015.12.010.

Woolcott, Orison O., Marilyn Ader, and Richard N. Bergman. 2015. "Glucose Homeostasis during Short-Term and Prolonged Exposure to High Altitudes." *Endocrine Reviews* 36 (2): 149–73. https://doi.org/10.1210/er.2014-1063.

Xu, Yan, Leslie R. Morse, Raquel Assed Bezerra da Silva, Paul R. Odgren, Hajime Sasaki, Philip Stashenko, and Ricardo A. Battaglino. 2009. "PAMM: A Redox Regulatory Protein That Modulates Osteoclast Differentiation." *Antioxidants & Redox Signaling* 13 (1): 27–37. https://doi.org/10.1089/ars.2009.2886.

Zheng, Jian Yong, Yi Gang Qiu, Dong Tao Li, Jiang Chun He, Yu Chen, Yi Cao, Ying Ming Liu, Xian Feng Li, Hai Tao Chi, and Tian Chang Li. 2017. "Prevalence and Composition of CHD at Different Altitudes in Tibet: A Cross-Sectional Study." *Cardiology in the Young* 27 (8): 1497–1503. https://doi.org/10.1017/S1047951117000567.

INDEX

A

Alagille syndrome, xi, 98, 103, 106, 107, 108, 109, 112, 113
Andean populations, 117, 120, 123, 125, 129, 159
Aortic Stenosis, 8, 20, 35, 36, 37
Atrial Septal Defect, v, viii, x, xi, xii, 3, 6, 20, 33, 79, 81, 83, 84, 85, 86, 87, 88, 89, 90, 91, 92, 94, 95, 98, 99, 101, 104, 107, 109, 116, 141, 142

B

birth defects, 2

C

cardiac resynchronization therapy, vii, ix, 56, 57, 58, 70, 71, 72
cardiogenic liver, xi, 98, 101
children, vi, viii, xi, xiii, 2, 6, 9, 21, 24, 67, 73, 84, 86, 95, 97, 98, 100, 103, 105, 109, 110, 111, 114, 116, 134, 141, 143, 144, 148, 177
chronic adaptation, 116, 118, 122, 159
Coarctation of the Aorta, 20, 38, 50, 167
congenital heart disease, vii, viii, ix, x, xi, 1, 2, 18, 19, 20, 21, 23, 24, 55, 56, 70, 71, 72, 73, 74, 79, 86, 97, 98, 99, 100, 101, 103, 109, 111, 113, 116, 134, 138, 177
coronary sinus atrial septal defects, xi, 80, 82

D

delivery plan, 30, 43

E

Ecuador, vi, viii, xii, xiii, 115, 116, 117, 138, 154, 155, 156, 158, 159, 160, 177, 178
Eisenmenger Syndrome, 35

F

Fontan, 17, 44, 45, 46, 59, 60, 66, 67, 69, 103, 111, 151, 183

H

heart failure, vii, viii, ix, xi, 5, 9, 13, 15, 18, 31, 34, 35, 37, 40, 41, 43, 46, 47, 55, 56, 57, 58, 59, 61, 67, 68, 69, 70, 73, 74, 84, 91, 92, 94, 98, 102, 110, 142

high altitude, viii, xi, xii, xiii, 116, 117, 118, 119, 120, 121, 122, 123, 124, 125, 126, 127, 128, 129, 130, 131, 132, 133, 134, 135, 137, 138, 139, 140, 141, 142, 143, 144, 145, 147, 150, 151, 154, 155, 158, 159, 177

high-risk pregnancy, 2

L

liver, vi, viii, xi, 45, 97, 98, 101, 102, 103, 106, 107, 108, 109, 110, 111, 124, 136

Lutembacher syndrome, 83

N

Native Americans, 117, 179

O

ostium primum, x, 6, 80, 81, 82, 83, 91, 93, 94

ostium primum atrial septal defect, 81, 83, 91, 93, 94

ostium secundum atrial septal defect, 80, 81, 83, 93

P

partial anomalous pulmonary venous return, 87

patent ductus arteriosus, xii, 2, 19, 34, 35, 99, 101, 104, 116, 136, 140, 141, 157, 167

postpartum, 3, 7, 15, 32, 41, 43, 45, 46, 47, 48, 144

preconception, vii, ix, 2, 16, 27, 28, 48

pregnancy, v, vii, viii, ix, xii, 1, 2, 3, 4, 5, 7, 8, 9, 10, 11, 12, 13, 14, 15, 16, 17, 18, 19, 20, 21, 22, 23, 24, 25, 26, 27, 28, 29, 32, 33, 34, 35, 36, 37, 38, 39, 40, 41, 43, 44, 45, 46, 48, 49, 50, 51, 52, 53, 99, 108, 116, 133, 134, 135, 176, 177, 180, 184

pulmonary hypertension, xii, 4, 5, 6, 7, 13, 17, 33, 35, 49, 81, 84, 94, 100, 101, 116, 120, 143, 144, 154

pulmonary stenosis, 19, 37, 38, 40, 148

S

septum primum, 7, 80, 83, 145

septum secundum, 80

severe left axis deviation, 86

sinus venosus, x, 6, 80, 81, 82, 87, 90, 93, 94, 95, 142

sinus venosus atrial septal defect, 82, 87, 90, 93, 94, 95

T

Tetralogy of Fallot, 12, 40, 148, 180

Transposition of the Great Vessels, 42, 140, 161

U

unroofed coronary sinus, 81, 83, 91, 93

V

Ventricular Septal Defect, viii, xi, 3, 4, 20, 34, 35, 98, 99, 109, 140, 143, 152

Related Nova Publications

THE REDISCOVERED TRICUSPID VALVE: STRUCTURE, FUNCTION AND CLINICAL SIGNIFICANCE IN HEALTH AND DISEASE

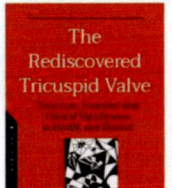

EDITOR: Giacomo Bianchi, MD, PhD

SERIES: Cardiology Research and Clinical Developments

BOOK DESCRIPTION: In order to better define the therapeutic path of a patient suffering from tricuspid valve disease, we have tried to offer a comprehensive overview to the reader, starting from historical considerations about the vision of the circulatory system and from the evidence accumulated over the centuries until the recognition of the continuum between signs and symptoms related to the valve.

HARDCOVER ISBN: 978-1-53616-098-7
RETAIL PRICE: $195

CONCEPTS, MATHEMATICAL MODELLING AND APPLICATIONS IN HEART FAILURE

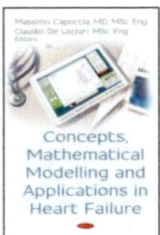

AUTHORS: Massimo Capoccia, MD, MSc Eng and Claudio De Lazzari, MSc Eng

SERIES: Cardiology Research and Clinical Developments

BOOK DESCRIPTION: Although there are probably enough publications about mechanical circulatory support, they do not seem to address the theoretical aspects with sufficient details. A more detailed knowledge of the interaction between ventricular assist devices (VADs) and the cardiovascular system may help with their clinical management with a view to improve patients' outcomes.

HARDCOVER ISBN: 978-1-53614-771-1
RETAIL PRICE: $230

To see a complete list of Nova publications, please visit our website at www.novapublishers.com

Related Nova Publications

A Closer Look at Cardiovascular Diseases and Risk Factors

Editor: Faris van Kilsdonk

Series: Cardiology Research and Clinical Developments

Book Description: In this compilation, the authors examine treatment options for this type of population. Bariatric surgery has proven to be an effective method, generating large weight reductions and improving cardiovascular risk factors, thus increasing the life expectancy of patients who undergo it.

Softcover ISBN: 978-1-53613-939-6
Retail Price: $95

Everything You Need to Know: Out of the Operating Room and Minimally Invasive Cardiothoracic Procedures

Editors: Dalia Banks, M.D. and Ahmed Zaky, M.D.

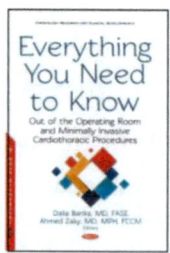

Series: Cardiology Research and Clinical Developments

Book Description: Being the first of its kind, this book is geared to meet and adapt to the rapidly expanding changes in the field of cardiothoracic surgery and anesthesia.

Hardcover ISBN: 978-1-53612-917-5
Retail Price: $230

To see a complete list of Nova publications, please visit our website at www.novapublishers.com